THE PROGRAM

21 DAYS TO A STRONGER, SLIMMER, SEXIER YOU

JESSIE PAVELKA

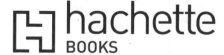

hachette
BOOKS

NEW YORK   BOSTON

Copyright © 2016 by Rowan Tree Fitness, Inc.
All interior photographs © 2016 Bradford Rogne Photography

Jacket design by Marlyn Dantes
Jacket photograph © Bradford Rogne Photography
Author photograph © Bradford Rogne Photography
Cover copyright © 2016 by Hachette Book Group, Inc.

Hachette Books
Hachette Book Group
1290 Avenue of the Americas
New York, NY 10104
HachetteBookGroup.com

First U.S. Edition: May 2016

Hachette Books is a division of Hachette Book Group, Inc.
The Hachette Books name and logo is a trademark of Hachette Book Group, Inc.

The publisher is not responsible for websites (or their content) that are not owned by the publisher.

The Hachette Speakers Bureau provides a wide range of authors for speaking events. To find out more, go to www.hachettespeakersbureau.com or call (866) 376-6591.

Library of Congress Cataloging-in-Publication Data

Names: Pavelka, Jessie, author.
Title: The program : 21 days to a stronger, slimmer, sexier you / by Jessie Pavelka.
Description: New York, NY : Hachette Books, [2016] | Includes index.
Identifiers: LCCN 2016001578| ISBN 9780316266567 (hardback) | ISBN 9781478909316 (audio download) | ISBN 9781478964919 (audio cd) | ISBN 9780316266536 (ebook)
Subjects: LCSH: Weight loss—Popular works. | Exercise—Popular works. | Weight loss—Psychological aspects—Popular works. | Self-care, Health—Popular works. | BISAC: HEALTH & FITNESS / Weight Loss.
Classification: LCC RM222.2 .P38 2016 | DDC 613.2/5—dc23 LC record available at http://lccn.loc.gov/2016001578

ISBNs: 978-0-316-26656-7 (hardcover), 978-0-316-26654-3 (paperback), 978-0-316-26653-6 (ebook)

Printed in the United States of America

RRD-C

10 9 8 7 6 5 4 3 2 1

*The Program is dedicated to everyone who decides
to take that first step toward something greater.
You'll never know how many lives you are changing.*

Table of Contents

Introduction

My work as a trainer gives me the privilege of helping people take charge of their bodies and lives. It is powerful to witness overweight and unhappy clients become confident, fit people. I have helped thousands of people reach many different goals and have realized that true fitness is not simply physical and can't be measured only by numbers on a scale. People who commit to improving their health not only get in better physical shape; they often become more optimistic and engaged partners, parents, and friends. They're inspiring. They're game. They're fun. Most of us are just plain happier when we're healthy.

It is a gift to see the impact of fitness not only on the individual, but on the people who love and care about them. I'm moved when I run into formerly sedentary clients with their children in the park, and see them climbing the jungle gym or riding on bicycles together. It's easier to make healthy choices and take care of yourself when you're happier. The amazing part is that people can make profound and dramatic improvements in their lives by taking a few small steps, over and over. Anyone can take them: move more, eat well, be mindful, and connect with others. That's it, that's everything, and this book is going to show you how to do it right.

Sports and exercise have defined and saved my life. I grew up in and around Corpus Christi, Texas, and spent most of my childhood playing outdoors. Farms, fields, the beach, gardens of bluebonnets: if it was outside, I was messing around in it, working up a sweat. As a good Texas boy, I rooted for the Cowboys and played football from the time I was four years old. Football was my favorite, but I enjoyed sports in general and played baseball and basketball and ran track through high school. As I got older and became intentional about shaping my own body for sport-specific performance in different seasons, I started spending more time in gyms and found myself learning a lot about training. I also found that people wanted to talk about this stuff with me and be able to do what I was doing. Eventually I realized that I could make some money this way, and I got professionally certified as a trainer when I was 19. I've worked with a lot of clients since then and figured out a thing or two about what I consider true fitness and how to get it. That's why I've created The Program. The Program will help you lose weight if you need to, but it's not a diet: it's a practical guide to living well that you can follow forever to be the strongest, happiest, best version of yourself.

People start training for many different reasons and need different strategies to reach their goals. Some clients are already pretty fit and want to take things to the next level or train for a specific sport or event. Other clients have been starting from tough places, maybe recovering from injury or illness, or they have a significant amount of weight to lose in order to get healthy. I designed The Program to be flexible so it can be used by anyone, at any fitness level, in an ongoing way.

You'll take action in four main areas on The Program—what you eat, how you move, mindfulness practices, and connecting with others—but you have a lot of freedom and flexibility to determine what makes you successful. You'll find a number of different ways to measure your progress as you move through The Program, and you can choose which ones feel most relevant to your life right now. You can choose different tools for measurement if and when your goals change. I've designed a cycle of workouts for three different levels of fitness that allow you to improve different areas of your performance and get some momentum without getting injured. The Program meal plan gives you the tools to choose foods that complement the kind of workout you're doing on any given day and that work for you and your family. There are multiple mindfulness practices you can try during the first cycle of The Program. You can incorporate the ones that are most motivating for you into your routine over the long haul. Creating relationships that feed your soul is a critical part of living well and directly impacts your physical fitness. I hope that the tools offered in The Program help you to begin, or strengthen, key relationships in your life. So, while The Program is a 21-day cycle, it has been designed for people at all different starting points with an understanding that our journeys to fitness never really end.

A lot of what I know about getting healthy is informed and inspired by my work with clients who have been seriously overweight. I've learned so much from their journeys. Sometimes I'm asked about how I found myself working so often with people who want to lose extreme amounts of weight. Here's what happened. I was living in California in my early twenties and developed a business called Fit for You with a friend and trainer named David Ryla. We created Fit for You to specialize in weight loss and work with bariatric patients who were preparing for, or recovering from, weight loss surgery. Now, my first clients as a trainer in Texas were generally people I had met in my own gym, and most of them were not overweight. The majority of them were already pretty fit and just wanting to get in better shape for themselves or their spouses, put on a little bit of muscle, or hit a performance goal for a specific sport. I was instinctively knowledgeable about a lot of that and enjoyed helping people reach those goals. The training experience with the Fit for You clients was very different. They were training because they wanted to live. Literally. Most of them were more than 100 pounds overweight and many had developed medical problems because of it. Someone who is facing bariatric surgery has gotten so out of shape that a doctor has told them they needed to get more fit, one way or another, in order to keep breathing.

When a person comes into the gym knowing it's a do-or-die situation, they usually work out with a special intensity. While they generally have a long road ahead of them, they also tend to see improvements very quickly. It is an amazing feeling to watch that person increase from three reps of an exercise to 12 reps or go from walking for 10 minutes to being able to run a mile without stopping. The confidence someone experiences in that situation is as inspiring to me as the weight they are losing or the strength they are building. Helping people discover, or rediscover, pride in their bodies and hope in their lives made me feel like I was not just doing work I enjoyed, but work that had the potential to be genuinely meaningful.

In addition to getting a great sense of satisfaction from training this new population, I was also getting a practical education about issues specific to clients dealing with extreme weight loss. In some ways, being heavy can strengthen your bones and help you develop certain muscles, but moving extra weight is hard work and tough on the body. My focus with very overweight people is always to protect their knees and feet at first, because that's where they are most vulnerable physically. They'll stop before they've barely started if they get injured in particular ways. I learned to use elliptical machines, the recumbent bike, swimming, and exercises for core balance and stability—less-weight-bearing activities that still got results.

At the same time I got a real education about other aspects of the physical side of this level of transformation, like pain and loose skin, as well as the psychological challenges involved in changing entrenched behavior patterns and family relationships. I had to learn how to keep people motivated when they are stalled and how to support them in developing and maintaining better eating habits. The stakes were high. It was challenging, stimulating, rewarding work. My experience with these clients inspired me to make movement a fundamental aspect of The Program. Being active increases your metabolism, provides a range of critical health benefits immediately even when your weight is not optimal, and keeps you motivated. So I like to get people moving right away. It helps if you can find a type of movement that you actually enjoy, but sometimes you need to reach a certain level of fitness before you can truly determine what movement suits you.

Even though I have not struggled with my own weight, I connected very personally with the Fit for Life clients when they talked about the ways that they had been using food to deal with unhappy feelings. It reminded me of the unhealthy behaviors I have used in my own life, with a similar lack of consciousness, to avoid my feelings. I could understand how hard it is to give up what you've come to rely upon so heavily, and how tough it can be to switch to healthier solutions, even when they make total sense. This empathy has served me well in working with clients, and perhaps especially so in working with those who need to lose an extreme amount of weight.

I became a professional trainer while I was still in college. Those years were a time of transition for me, as they are for so many people. I had been admitted to the University of North Texas as a starting fullback on their football team and began attending workouts with that team just a month or so after graduating high school. But I had broken my scapula a few years earlier and was experiencing some problems from that old injury. Long story short, I had to quit the team. And, believe me, I know it would sound cooler if we were talking about the NFL, but I had no idea what a big impact it would have on me to stop playing.

As a young man without football, I was lost. I didn't understand that I had a life-long relationship with football, and I had no idea how to deal with the sadness that would follow when I had to give it up. Sports had played a huge role for me, psychologically, as I was growing up. When I struggled with emotional things as a kid, such as my parents' divorce when I was nine, playing sports had allowed me to channel a lot of uncomfortable feelings of loss and powerlessness, even if I wasn't consciously aware of that at the time. All of a sudden, that outlet was gone. Finally, and this is no small thing: the routines and demands of being a four-season student athlete had provided the daily structure for most of my life up to that point. I suddenly found myself with a lot of time on my hands and didn't always make great choices about how to spend it.

Now, I could not have explained any of this to you—or to myself—as a college freshman. And I didn't really try to talk about my feelings with anyone at the time, as so many of us don't. But I was struggling. I coped, in part, by doing what I knew best: working out. I was already a regular user of weights and I continued to go to the gym every day, which kept me somewhat sane and safe. Exercise kept me grounded, and I started to focus more on bodybuilding. I got into power moves: dead lifts, bench press, power clean. These were all things I had done before, with particular goals for getting bigger, stronger, and faster in particular ways for specific sports or games. But without a sport to train for, my goal in the gym just became to get bigger and stronger, period. There was no end in sight, no sense of "Here is where I'm happy, here is where I stop."

When I look back on that time, I know that even though I was fit and strong, I was working out in a way that became unhealthy. And I can see that I was also kind of grieving, although I didn't regret the decision to stop playing football. It was just that I had to deal with my life for the first time without letting a sport distract me, and I didn't know how to do that. I guess my response was just to focus on the outside part of me. In addition to connecting with a lot of people at the gym who shared my enthusiasm for exercise, I also joined a fraternity. I made good friends there, and it replaced some of that team-like camaraderie I was used to, but without the stabilizing factor of sport. I was working out hard, socializing intensely, and was often exhausted.

I was getting a lot of good feedback about how strong I was becoming. The owner of the gym I worked out in encouraged me to try a bodybuilding competition. My girl-friend at the time had already done one, so she offered to help me train for it. Always up for a challenge, I enjoyed the process of training for a competition and learning how people can use weights and exercise to precisely manipulate their muscles and body composition to control how they look. It was different from the way I had worked out before, and it felt good to have a purpose driving my gym time again. But the competition itself, with the music and the posing trunks and choreography parts of it—that just felt uncomfortable to me! Maybe it's being a guy from Texas, I don't know, but I didn't like it, and I knew that even though I'd placed second, I'd never do another one. I guess everything happens for a reason, though, because that one competition got me noticed by Ed Connors, who was based in California and owned Gold's Gym. Ed called me up one day after seeing that competition and said something like, "You have a future in fitness or bodybuilding," and offered me a job.

It did not take a lot of convincing to get me to move from Denton, Texas, to Palm Desert, California. I knew that I needed a change. I was partying about as hard as I was training, which I sensed was not sustainable. And I was ready for new challenges.

Over the next few years, I experimented with different types of training techniques and fitness activities with a variety of clients; connected with other professionals who shared my interests; started Fit for You and learned about running a small business; began exploring other aspects of health, including nutrition and mindfulness practices; and helped build a gym. I was also still working out hard on my own and starting to do magazine features and covers in fitness industry magazines, like *Muscle & Fitness* and *Maximum Fitness.* Most trainers who do this are naturally pursuing it in order to promote a brand or a product, but I was still pretty young and treating it almost as a little hobby or side sport. It took me a while, but I learned a lot about creating successful strategies for training different types of clients, developed an understanding of the fitness industry as a whole, and figured out the kinds of things that help me maintain some balance in my own life and create a vision for my future.

As you might guess, gyms are meaningful places to me. Exercise has been my anchor. When I go to the gym, life is just not that bad. Using my body helps to remind me that I'm alive and sometimes it allows emotion to move around a bit and come to the front of my brain and release itself in unexpected ways. One of the things I've learned from my clients is how we wear emotions in different parts of our bodies and that exercise can allow us to release it. If you want to help someone find a way to get to the core of a problem, get them moving: when someone is exhausted, all those filters we put in place to protect ourselves drop away and the truth emerges. Gaining weight, for many of the people I work with, was a slow process of avoiding dealing with uncomfortable feelings. Once you acknowledge what you have been trying to bury you can start to deal with it directly.

Listening to my clients changed my training methods. I began paying more attention to the mind-body connection, started understanding the difference between changing the body for health versus appearance, and developed a deeper appreciation for the spiritual side of exercise.

Sometimes I think we start the day off strong, at full power, and as we move through it, we have interactions that drain us of our power and commitment: we run late, our kids give us a hard time, our boss is in a bad mood, we get bad news in the mail, something in the house breaks. It doesn't matter what it is, but stuff happens that distracts and depletes us and all of a sudden, many of us make unhealthy choices without even thinking about it. The Program incorporates strategies to help you harness your mind power throughout each day. You can use specific techniques at any moment to stay calm and centered, and remind yourself about what is really important and how you want to live. These techniques include journaling, meditation, and breathing exercises that are simple but truly effective for staying disciplined. They will also help you stay committed to your fitness path.

The Program is going to teach you how to eat more mindfully, with an awareness of when and how to fuel your body for maximum performance and health. The mindfulness techniques I'll be asking you to try can benefit anyone in a variety of ways, but they have been especially useful for my clients who have a history of eating or drinking in order to avoid feeling bad or bored or frustrated. It's not a magic bullet, of course, but being intentionally conscious about what you feel, and when and why you want to eat, usually helps people make better choices about food. The mindfulness practices also help many of my clients realize how much better they feel when they move more.

While I love the gym, there is also something special to me about exercising outdoors and I'll be encouraging you to get outside during The Program. Hiking is one of my favorite activities. It's great because you're moving, but there is also the possibility of a sense of connection to something greater than yourself. If you are moved by watching an amazing sunset, it might just be because it's beautiful, I don't know, but I'd like to think there's something else going on there. It's a moment when you can say, "Are my issues really that significant when you look at this sky?" Nature is an expression of God for me; it is both grounding and inspirational. I spent a lot of time at the beach with my family when I was growing up, because we were near the Gulf of Mexico, and getting out near the Pacific Ocean is one of my favorite parts of living in California. There is probably a landscape that you find especially meaningful or inspirational, and if there isn't, maybe you'll discover one as you begin moving and exploring more outside.

Wherever you wind up liking to exercise, you may find that in addition to making you physically stronger, working out can be a time when you get very creative. I find that I can get a flow going on a hike or at the gym that is almost meditative. It's a head space where I can really sort things out. Working out reminds me that some things might be wrong but I have this capable body. Appreciating something so basic can buoy your spirits right there. It also feels great: when I leave the gym after a hard workout, I am buzzing from the serotonin and dopamine my body releases. You don't have to be interested in understanding the chemical process to know when you just feel good, and I promise that you can't help but feel good when you give yourself the gift of movement and exercise. You'll also find that feeling good helps you make positive choices around the food you cook and eat.

Feeling good about yourself also makes it easier to have relationships with other people who can support you on your journey and remind you of your purpose. Many people I work with who are trying to lose a lot of weight have really isolated themselves. It's hard to stay connected to others when you're feeling unhappy and dissatisfied with yourself. I know that I make stronger, healthier decisions when I'm actively checking in with my family, especially my parents and my sisters. That's one of the reasons that being connected to people who care about you—whether they are actual blood relatives or not—is a key part of The Program. Don't be tempted to skip over that section of The Program if you're excited to get started and it doesn't seem like your relationships are directly related to fitness or weight loss. I have learned from my clients and in my own life that true fitness emanates from both inside and outside the body. Connecting with others helps you get and stay there.

Don't be alarmed if that piece of The Program is a new one for you. It's important to try stepping out of your comfort zone. Working on this book has been rewarding but also challenging for me: writing is a real change of lens in my world, where physical exercise has always been easy. It's okay—even good!—if some aspects of The Program are more challenging for you than others. We don't change without being challenged. And it's okay to be flat-out scared. One of my favorite things to do on some of the television shows I've worked on is to have people try a fitness activity that forces them to face some sort of personal anxiety. Sometimes it's water, sometimes it's heights—it doesn't matter: the exhilaration someone experiences after conquering their fear is contagious and inspiring. Many times, a person's fear is not so specific, but more a general kind of distrust about whether or not they can really get healthy and fit. I don't have to know anything about you to know that it's possible to improve your fitness, that how far you can go requires challenging yourself, and that your effort will be worth it. Once you decide you're going to do something, and you've done your homework so you know it's safe, try to get out of your own way and just dive in and try it. I've done a lot of the homework for you. Sometimes I tell people I work with "Don't think too much, just jump off the cliff." It's not the most gentle approach, and I guess it's my own version of feel the fear and do it anyway. But, really, once you make a decision, acknowledge the doubt and jump. Give yourself a chance to be surprised.

Maybe you have tried to lose weight before and it didn't go so well. Or maybe it went really well but you gained it all back. That's common. Almost any reasonable diet will work when you're following it, but most of them aren't realistic or flexible enough to stay on for the long term. Fundamentally, your weight is only one component of your fitness. If you can make a commitment to eat, sweat, think, and connect every day with hope and intention, you're going to become more fit in every way that matters, and you'll feel better. You might even think about your weight loss as a kind of happy side effect of treating yourself well.

It takes conscious effort to make permanent changes to live well, and The Program will show you how to do it. If you've picked up this book, you probably aren't exactly where you want to be right now. You might be scared to start or fail. It's okay. If this is you, I don't care how out of shape or unhappy you are: I promise that things are not as bad as they seem. You can make changes, and it doesn't have to be a big thing. It can happen right now. This may feel like jumping off a cliff, but it's only some simple things we're talking about: Get up and get moving. Believe in yourself and be hopeful. Do the work. Focus on taking action that will make you feel good in your own skin today. You're not just going to chase a distant goal, although it's fine to set one. But if you take the actions I lay out in The Program, you are going to feel better right now. And this all gets easier as time passes. The longer you stick with The Program, the stronger you'll be.

Making healthy choices over the long haul gets easier because you develop good habits and self-discipline, but it also requires constantly renewing your motivation. I'm a father now, and it has changed my life in every imaginable way. My son, Rowan, causes me to look at so many aspects of life differently, from being more concerned about the quality of the food we eat and the environment we live in to a renewed consciousness about the larger impact of my own actions and decisions. Rowan is only six, and already I can see how fast our time together is moving. He makes me want to really be present and appreciate every moment we have together. Just hanging out with him, whether we're playing outside, building with Legos, or drawing together, is an inspirational reminder of why I want to be the healthiest, strongest, best version of myself for as long as I possibly can.

Enough about me already! It's time to think about your Why. This book has your How covered and it's going to be easier than you think. As you follow The Program, you'll be focusing on:

Eating nutritious, delicious food. You are going to eat whole foods that fuel your workouts, promote your health, and make you feel good.

Moving more. You're going to build your strength and endurance, improve your agility and flexibility, boost your metabolism, and feel more comfortable in your body.

Living mindfully. You are going to take a few minutes each day to breathe, relax, reflect, and remind yourself of what you want and how much you already have.

Connecting with people who care about you. You are going to cultivate some key relationships—including the one you have with yourself—that will help sustain and inspire you to be your best self.

When you do these things, your body will get faster and stronger than it is right now. You will sleep better at night and be energized and empowered as you move through your day. You are going to have more patience and compassion for the people around you. Yes, if you follow The Program you are going to look better. But, more important, you are probably going to be happier. You are just plain going to feel good. The best part is there is no end in sight because you can use The Program for the rest of your life. Let's get started.

Goals

SETTING GOALS AND STAYING MOTIVATED

One of the best parts of my job is being able to see people reach their goals. The goals of the people I've worked with have varied tremendously. Some of my clients, at all different kinds of weights and fitness levels, have been miserable and depressed, and felt that being healthier would help them feel happier, find love, find more fulfilling work, or be better parents to their children. Other very overweight clients had been quite satisfied and happy with their lives, but came to me when they were faced with a health crisis and they needed to get healthier in order to avoid a massive sacrifice in the quality of their lives.

There are times when people's goals are very personal. I worked with a sweet woman who had always loved horses and lived on a farm but had gotten to 420 pounds and could no longer do much of anything. She had limited mobility and was deeply depressed. Feeding and caring for her horses was just about the only form of physical activity she engaged in: the rest of the day was spent sitting on her couch. Her goal was to be able to ride a horse again. So we burned that couch—literally!—and set our goal to get her to a weight at which she could safely ride a horse and start engaging in life again, then take it from there. She reached that milestone at 290 pounds. I don't know what your Why is, but one thing I've learned is that figuring out what it is and keeping that Why in the forefront of your mind is the key to living a healthy, well-balanced life. In the same way that our Whys can vary, so can the ways we measure progress as we move toward our goals.

You need to set some goals. Let's say you want to lose weight. I don't know what you weigh now, what you want to weigh, or how long it will take you to get from here to there, based on your current fitness level. Here's what I do know: You can get there. You will enjoy the journey more than you think you're going to. It will probably be slower than you think it's going to be and your progress may not be consistent. It will be easier to keep faith with yourself if you track your progress. There are a bunch of acceptable ways to do that.

THE SCALE

I'll be honest: I personally don't use a scale. I know that might sound funny in light of my work on *The Biggest Loser*, and I know many people find them to be a useful tool. So if that's you, go ahead and weigh yourself. After you establish your starting weight, put that thing away for 2 weeks—1 week if you can't stand it. But, really no less than that, because your weight will fluctuate a bit from day to day for a bunch of different reasons and you don't want to get demoralized over a number that reflects that you just drank a lot of water or something. Weighing yourself once a week, or every 2 weeks, will be a more accurate reality check and be less apt to drive you crazy. Keep two things in mind if this is how you are going to measure your progress. First, it will be most accurate if you weigh yourself under the same conditions each time you do it (at the same time of day and wearing the same type of clothing). Second, if you are building more lean muscle mass, the scale may not reflect some real progress because muscle weighs more than fat. There may be times when you worked hard for a week, really improved your mood and body in a variety of ways, and yet see a number on the scale that is disappointing to you. It can be a true test of character to push through that, but some people get discouraged by it, and there are other legitimate ways of assessment.

BODY MEASUREMENTS

It takes more time to measure key body parts than it does to step on the scale, but it is another valid way to track changes in your body. This method can be very encouraging, since you will usually feel positive about one or more of the measurements even if another one is disappointing. You can measure your chest, arms, waist, hips, thighs, and calves using an ordinary soft tape measure. Don't take these measurements more than once every 2 weeks.

If you want to do this, be as precise as you can, but don't stress too much. As long as you keep your measuring methods consistent from week to week, you'll be tracking changes in your body accurately. For all the measurements, keep the tape measure parallel to the floor and flat on your body without pressing too hard.

Arms: Place the tape measure all the way around the widest part of your arm above the elbow (the middle of the biceps).

Calves: While you're standing up, place the tape measure around the widest point of your calves.

Hips: Place the tape measure around the widest point of your hips, right across your hip bones and buttocks.

Thighs: Place the tape measure around the widest point of your thigh.

Waist: Place the tape measure all the way around your torso around your natural waist, about an inch above your bellybutton. Don't suck in your stomach!

Chest: Place the tape measure all the way around the fullest part of your chest, across your nipples.

For some people, recording these six numbers every few weeks provides motivating feedback on their progress.

CLOTHES

Do you have a pair of pants or a dress that you would like to fit into (or back into)? Try them on once a week and watch yourself get closer to your goal. You know this is a reality check because many of us start to notice if we have gained weight when our ordinary pants start to feel tight. This works best if the item is fairly fitted (for example, a pair of jeans or a size 8 dress) and made out of a constructed fabric as opposed to a loosely sized (S-M-L) garment made from a stretchy fabric or with an elastic in the waistband. One other thing: if your motivational clothing item is a whole lot smaller than you currently are, keep it to inspire you but consider getting something else you like within, let's say, two or three sizes of your current size. Use that as a subgoal size to measure your progress. Some people find this to be a concrete and satisfying form of motivation and reward.

BODY FAT PERCENTAGE

This one requires going to a gym or a doctor or getting your hands on some equipment, because I'm guessing you don't have calipers or other types of body composition analysis in your house. But these tools exist, with varying degrees of accuracy, and you can have an assessment done if that appeals to you, then have it repeated on a regular basis. Make sure the follow-up is done using the same method you used for the baseline measurement. How often you have this done will vary depending on the method you use, but it should be at least once a month. If you're having a body fat percentage evaluation less frequently, use this in combination with another method as well.

EXERCISE ASSESSMENTS

Pick a few—let's say four—exercises (you could use ones from the assessment tests on The Program) and record your progress every week. You could see how many push-ups, sit-ups, or burpees you can do in 60 seconds, and then time how long you can hold a plank or a wall sit. You could also time how long it takes you to walk or run a mile. Whichever exercises you choose, you can practice them as part of your regular workout routine, then do the timed tests once a week. These can be very motivating, because, like the body measurements, you'll almost always have some encouraging result in one area if you are disappointed in another. It's also a nice way of reminding yourself of how much stronger you are getting.

THE FEEL-GOOD SCALE

Are you a numbers person? Try looking beyond the number of pounds on the scale. There are four main elements to The Program: you will Eat, Sweat, Think, and Connect in a mindful way that promotes your health every day. At the end of each day, consider your actions in each of these areas, and if you want to give yourself a score, try this:

Eat: Did each of your main meals follow the recommended food portions and exchanges for the day? Give yourself 1 point for each meal that hit your target (total possible = 3 points).

Sweat: Did you do both workouts today? Give yourself 1 point for each one you completed (total possible = 2 points).

Think: Did you set an intention, take a moment to breathe, try a mindfulness activity, and record three grateful or happy moments? Give yourself 1 point for each opportunity you took to be mindful (total possible = 4 points).

Connect: I'll be asking you to work on four key relationships during The Program, but, unlike the mindfulness activities, most of this work takes more than a few minutes, so I don't expect you to do something for each relationship every day. But I do ask you to take one daily action in pursuit of connection. Did you do one thing today to connect in a healthy way to yourself, a higher power, other people, or the wider world? Did you touch base with your accountability partner? Did you take a new class? Did you go for a bike ride with your child? Walk in nature? Call your mom? Give yourself 1 point if you connected with someone (total possible = 1 point).

That's a somewhat arbitrary 10-point scale. Some people find themselves very motivated by a number, and if wanting that tenth point helps remind you to take a moment to set an intention in the morning, use it. If you score a 10, I bet you'll be feeling like the day treated you pretty well, and it'll be because you took actions that encouraged that outcome. If you find you're consistently scoring lower than a 10, look at your patterns to see where you can try different strategies.

HOW DO YOU FEEL?

This is a variation of the Feel-Good Scale but without the point system. It is still an intentional assessment. Take some time each week to reflect on your progress. You can write this down, but you don't have to. How did you do this week? Ask yourself all the same questions you would if you were using the Feel-Good Scale and just consider what is working and not working and whether there is anything you can do to troubleshoot in the places that you're stumbling, and reward yourself for what is going well. Think about how you are feeling. Are you happier? Calmer? More energized? Think about your Why. Do you feel like you're making progress toward that goal?

STAYING MOTIVATED

You are going to have moments where you don't want to exercise, even though you know it's good for you and even though you know you are going to feel better after you do it. Everyone needs motivation—even me sometimes. But I've found that if you take the body, the mind will follow. Tell yourself you can do 5 minutes. Put your sneakers on, commit to 5 minutes, and do it. That 5 minutes will almost always turn into more time, and you'll be glad you did it. It's really that simple.

Sometimes I have clients who feel motivated to work out and are working hard, but get discouraged because they hit a plateau in their weight loss. The reality is that the body adapts to new routines quickly, and when this happens, it may be a message that you need to do a little more. When I troubleshoot with people in this situation, we make sure that they're clear and realistic about what they have been eating and how much they've been moving, and often we'll find that something has gone off track. But when someone has truly been sticking to their plan and is no longer seeing it translate in numbers on the scale, I try to help people look at this potentially frustrating moment as a kind of gift. Even a moment for celebration. You are graduating to a new phase of your training, where you can take on more responsibility and push the boundaries of your potential. If you've been walking, maybe you're ready to run. That's an amazing moment.

The toughest times are when it's just you, alone, surrounded by potentially bad choices with no trainer to perform for, no fans in the stands, and no accountability partner. You have to challenge yourself to be the best, most powerful version of yourself at those times and remind yourself about why you're doing this. Knowing that it's not all about the scale helps people stay motivated.

Eat

Food is fuel. Athletes don't diet, they eat, and there is a direct correlation between nutrition and performance. The food that I'm recommending you eat on The Program will help you meet your nutritional needs, maximize your performance when you work out, aid your digestion, and improve your health and your mood. If your diet is a typical American one right now, you're going to lose weight over the next few weeks if you follow my plan. And you are definitely going to feel better.

There are a lot of weight loss plans out there that will tell you that a calorie is a calorie, no matter where it comes from. The reality is that everything you eat affects your blood chemistry, and in the same way that you want to be doing high-performance training to get the most out of your workouts, you want to do high-performance eating. Most, if not all, of the food you eat should be nutritionally dense with a sense of purpose to increase your power. This means that most processed foods, which have generally been stripped of their nutrients, vitamins, and minerals, are no longer going to have a place in your cabinets and on your table. It's not only what's missing from these foods but how your body processes them that's problematic. The white flour and sugar that make up such a big part of most packaged foods increase the enzymes that promote inflammation in the body, which is associated with so many disease risks.

In addition to cutting down on processed foods, you know what you need to do: cut back on sugar, eat more vegetables, and drink more water. This is good basic strategy for weight loss, and you'll be following it on The Program. But we're taking it to the next level, because I don't want you to eat just to lose weight. I want you to eat whole, real, powerhouse foods in combinations that fuel your inner athlete and help you become healthy and well. I've paired specific menu plans with specific types of workouts to help you optimize your performance, boost your metabolism, and promote your health. The bottom line is that what you eat and how you move can keep your insulin levels under control, decrease inflammation in your body, and make you feel good. There are properties in specific foods, spices, and herbs that can optimize your body for health, and The Program is going to help you incorporate them into your diet, too.

TAKING CHARGE

Experts tell us that our eating habits in the United States are improving. As a nation, the number of calories we eat every day has gone down a bit. And obesity rates are stabilizing. This is all good news. But we can do better. Two-thirds of adult Americans are overweight, and more than a third are obese. About a third of school-age children in the United States are overweight, as are about 25 percent of children under age five. The problem has intensified during my lifetime: all of these numbers are at least twice what they were in the 1970s.

The standard American diet has more saturated fat, salt, added sugar, and refined grains than experts tells us are healthy and less than the recommended amounts of vegetables, fruit, whole grains, and dairy. Did you start your day with a bowl of breakfast cereal or a bagel with juice and coffee, follow up with a meat and cheese sandwich on white bread with chips for lunch, then have a couple slices of pizza for dinner with a side salad? If so, you have a lot of company. And you can do—and feel—so much better.

Most of us don't work up a sweat often enough, either. Are you moving for at least 30 minutes every day? Only about 5 percent of Americans do. Only about a third of adult Americans are getting the recommended amount of exercise each week for their age group, and about a quarter of adults report being completely inactive. The numbers aren't great for kids in the United States either: only one in three are physically active every day and our children are spending an average of 7 hours a day in front of some kind of screen.

You know why this is a problem. When you don't move enough and eat more than you need to, you're likely to wind up overweight. Being overweight puts you at an increased risk for heart disease, diabetes, and certain kinds of cancer, among other things. It lowers your mortality in the long term. It is likely to increase your medical costs. And if you are carrying more weight than you need, you probably just plain don't feel your best day to day. Now, it's possible to be overweight and relatively fit. Only you know where you are and where you want to be in terms of your weight. But 60 percent of us say we want to weigh less, which makes sense given those statistics.

The Program can help you do that, but this isn't just about you getting skinny. The Program is about you getting strong, being healthy, and feeling well in your body—for the rest of your life.

WHAT YOU EAT

Eating on The Program means eating mindfully. It means paying attention to the ratio of lean protein, good carbohydrates, and healthy fat in the foods you eat, and I'm going to make it very easy for you to figure out how to do that, so that you can use my recipes and meal plans or swap out foods with things that work for you and your family. There is no category of food that is completely off limits, but I've provided lists of better choices within major food categories that you can use to make your own decisions. As you assess the way you feel when you are eating to promote your health and performance, I'm betting it will get easier and easier to make the best choices.

Eating mindfully on The Program also means paying attention to when you eat. Don't worry, I'm not going to tell you have to eat at a particular time of day or that you can't eat certain food groups after breakfast or anything like that. The Program is meant to fit into your life the way you want to live it. But this is also your new life, one that involves moving, as a commitment to yourself and your well-being. To optimize your workouts, you want to think about how you are going to sweat each day and when you're going to do it, because that is going to help you make your best eating choices.

There are four different types of Eat days on The Program: Cleanse, Burn, Build, and Relax. During the next few weeks, you're going to follow them in the order that I've developed here, but once you complete this cycle and have the hang of eating this way—which will happen quickly—you can just choose your days as they work best for you. You will never need to leave The Program to eat "normally" or get bored following one routine endlessly because it's very flexible.

Cleanse: This is not a "detox" or a "cleanse" in the sense that you have probably heard those terms before (more about that later). On a Cleanse day, you're going to eat light, eat clean, and give your digestive system a bit of a break. You'll be eating nutrient-rich smoothies and soups that will reset your palate. This is not a fast, and you will not be hungry. The recipes I'm recommending for these particular days use foods that have some evidence-based properties for healing the body and strengthening the immune system in various ways. I call them the Core Four ingredients, and you can incorporate them into your diet during other days as well if you like how they make you feel. You'll start The Program with four Cleanse eating days to prime your body for what is to come.

Burn: You are going to move more on The Program, and you need to fuel yourself properly with the right ratio of complex carbohydrates to protein. You'll be eating slightly more carbohydrates on the Burn days, and you can tailor the meal plans depending on the time of day you train so that you can get the most out of your workouts. Certain types of protein are easier for your body to digest, as are particular combinations of macronutrients.

Build: Building muscle and getting strong are critical parts of The Program. You need protein every day (with every meal, actually), and eating the right kind and amount of protein after strength training helps your muscles repair and develop in an optimal way. You'll eat to build, feeding your muscles on the days that you focus on strength training. You can pay attention to when and what you're eating relative to when you work out in order to maximize the relationship between your food and your workout. Build days have slightly more protein compared with the days that you're doing Burn workouts.

Relax: I struggled with what to call this day, because I hope you'll be calm and relaxed most of the time on The Program, particularly in terms of your food. The body responds very quickly to being well nourished, and I think you're going to like how you feel. But this is a day when you relax your standards a little and allow yourself something you wouldn't normally have on The Program. There is not a recommended meal plan for a Relax day because I don't know what kind of food or drink you enjoy that needs to have a limited role in your healthy diet. But I know most of us have foods in that category. For me, it might be a burger and a beer! This is not a "cheat" meal or day; it's part of The Program that recognizes the realities of our lives and helps you plan for them and incorporate them into an eating plan that does not derail your hard work. You can—and should!—still train on your Relax eating day, and how you choose to do that will determine how you plan to eat that day. I've given you an example of what a Relax day might look like for me, so you can use it as a guide.

Here's what's going to happen: You're going to eat on the "Cleanse" schedule for 4 days to kick-start The Program, followed by eating in alternating Build-Burn cycles for the next 17 days. At the end of that, you'll experience a Relax eating day to understand what it looks like. This chart lays it out for you starting on a Sunday, but you don't have to begin The Program on any particular day of the week.

Sunday	Monday	Tuesday	Wednesday	Thursday	Friday	Saturday
Cleanse	Cleanse	Cleanse	Cleanse	Burn	Build	Burn
Build	Burn	Build	Burn	Build	Burn	Build
Burn	Build	Burn	Build	Burn	Build	Burn
Relax						

Once you've completed that cycle and adjusted to this way of eating, you can repeat it or adjust it as it suits you. I have clients who schedule a Cleanse eating day once a week as part of their routine, and other clients who only use a Cleanse day when they feel they need a bit of a reset. If you find that you are doing a lot of strength training, you may use the Build day eating plan more often. If you are primarily in a state of weight maintenance, you might allow yourself a Relax day more often than someone who is working hard to lose weight. The choice is yours, and the plan can be changed as your workouts change, as you grow stronger, and as your goals evolve.

The differences between your Cleanse, Burn, Build, and Relax days are subtle but real. They have to do with the ratio of carbohydrates to protein to fat in the meals you'll eat on those days, and when you eat them. Each type of eating day on The Program is designed with a PCF ratio in mind (the percentage of food you eat during the day that is made up of protein, carbohydrates, and fat), and you are going to start thinking about your overall diet in terms of these macronutrients.

Protein

Your body needs protein to supply amino acids that your body needs to build and repair muscle and make essential enzymes and hormones. You also need it for energy and a well-functioning immune system. The average American gets less than 20 percent of their daily calories as protein, most of it at dinner. That doesn't necessarily mean people aren't getting enough protein. You may or may not be meeting your minimum protein requirements (that depends on your size), but if you are eating too many fats and carbohydrates, the ratio of your nutrients will keep you from functioning in top form. The benefits of higher protein intake relative to carbohydrates and fats in your diet are huge: it will help you build and maintain a leaner body that burns fat more efficiently and help preserve muscle strength as you age. Most of you are going to be building muscle on The Program and will benefit from paying attention to your protein. Protein matters even if building muscle isn't your main goal: eating adequate protein and spacing it out over the day's meals and snacks will keep you feeling energized. After you complete the four Cleanse days, you are going to eat protein at every meal.

If you are trying to lose weight, research suggests that eating more protein helps you avoid losing lean muscle along with excess fat. Don't underestimate the satiety factor of protein-rich foods either: if you're getting used to eating less overall, protein will keep you feeling full, help reduce your appetite, and actually require your body to work a little harder to digest it, compared with fat or carbohydrates, which burns a few more calories. Many of my clients report being less likely to overeat in the protein category compared with carbohydrates and fat.

In addition to paying attention to how much protein you eat and when you eat it, you'll want to think about what type of protein you tend to eat. It's best if most of your protein is lean. If a lot of your protein has been coming from things like sausage, bacon, red meat, or processed deli meats, that's got to change. You will fuel more efficiently and maximize your nutrients if you vary your diet to incorporate leaner sources of protein like chicken, fish, turkey, beans, nuts, and whole grains. If you can eat dairy, remember that Greek yogurt, milk, eggs, and cheese can also be good protein sources. There are also high-quality protein supplements you can use in smoothies or to give other recipes a protein boost. Whey, egg, hemp, and pea-based supplements are my preference if you want to give these a try. Finally, since many (not all) of these protein sources have a better PCF ratio than beef, you can often eat more of them. Red meat does not have to be eliminated from your diet if you like it, but consider expanding your repertoire of protein foods on The Program.

Carbohydrates

I know it's trendy to cut carbohydrates if you're trying to lose weight, but, like protein, not all carbohydrate sources are the same, and the athlete in you can benefit from the good ones. Carbohydrates are the body's primary source of energy and are needed for the healthy functioning of your kidneys, intestines, brain, and central nervous system.

At this point, I'm thinking that you probably know what to do about carbohydrates if you're eating for health. You need to eat fewer carbohydrates that come in the form of sugar and refined flour, like white bread, rice, and pasta. That's not strictly about eating less, although you probably will if you cut way down on these foods, since they are so easy to overeat. It's really about the quality of white flour and sugar as energy sources: they're a quick source of energy but poor fuel. Refined carbohydrates trigger a large release of insulin in your body and get stored as extra fat when you don't use them. And they do seem easy for most people to overeat.

But you don't need to cut carbohydrates out of your diet in order to lose weight—and you shouldn't. Your muscles and your brain need glucose for energy, and you produce glucose when you digest carbohydrates. You want to choose more complex carbohydrates that your body will burn more slowly, and you want to try to eat them in combination with other foods that slow down their digestion. Complex carbohydrates—the kind you get in fruits and vegetables, whole grains, beans, nuts, seeds, milk, and yogurt—come with all kinds of vitamins, minerals, and other vital nutrients that are good for you. The fiber in most of them helps your digestive system function properly and makes you feel full, so you're likely to eat less. As a bonus, most nonstarchy vegetables and fruits are nutrient dense and relatively low in calories. If you commit to seriously increasing the amount of produce in your diet and making those your primary source of carbohydrates, I can almost guarantee you're going to start to eat fewer calories.

You can have complex carbohydrates at each meal or not—it's up to you. Your decisions can be made depending on when and how you're working out. When you choose healthy ones—like oats or quinoa—they will help you keep your blood sugar stable, take longer to digest, and come with their nutrients still intact. Just pay attention to the quantity you're eating and what you're eating them with.

Fat

You need to eat some fat. Period. It's another form of fuel—actually your most concentrated energy source. Certain forms of it can help reduce your risk for heart disease. It maintains the health of your cell membranes, skin, and hair, and is essential for some of your organs to function properly. Some key vitamins, like A, D, E, and K, are actually absorbed better with fat, so the nutritional benefits of the vegetables in a salad are actually improved by your using a little fat in the form of nuts, cheese, or dressing. Fat tends to help you feel satisfied as well: it makes food taste good, which is important, and you digest fat a bit more slowly than carbohydrates, so it should keep you feeling full.

Some people trying to lose weight get nervous about eating fat. It's true that fat tends to be more calorie dense than protein and carbohydrates (9 calories per gram compared with 4 calories per gram) so you do have to watch your portions. The good news is that a little usually goes a long way.

As with carbohydrates and protein, there are different types of fat, and you want to primarily get yours as unsaturated fat. Heart-healthy choices like olive oil, high-oleic sunflower or safflower oil, nuts, olives, avocados, and salmon should be the primary sources of fat in your diet. Saturated fats, which tend to be solid at room temperature and have saturated fatty acids, affect the level of cholesterol in your blood, both good and bad, and can have a limited place in most people's diets. I eat egg yolks and cook with coconut oil fairly regularly. You'll also find saturated fat in meat, butter, cream, cheese, and chocolate. Trans fats, which you are most likely to see in the form of partially hydrogenated oil, have been shown to increase your risk for heart disease and have no place in your body or on The Program. Trans fats are yet another reason to eliminate packaged snack foods and baked foods that are designed to be shelf stable from your diet!

The food choices you'll make on The Program should be driven by the combination of protein, carbohydrates, and fat in your meals and during each day. The types of foods you use to supply those macronutrients do matter, and I've created sample meal plans to suggest good choices, but you have a lot of flexibility within the categories to plan meals that work for you and your family.

Sugar

Scientists tell us that refined sugar is an addictive substance. I mean addictive in a similar sense to alcohol or cigarettes, with associated health consequences. When you eat sugar—and refined carbohydrates like white bread are processed in your body like sugar even if they don't taste sweet—your body experiences a rush and then a rapid depletion, like a drug high. Your blood sugar spikes and then your body releases insulin to help your cells absorb that sugar. When that happens, your blood sugar drops back down and your body wants that rush all over again. The whole process happens quickly, like a roller coaster. It creates stress and inflammation in the body and can leave you biochemically imbalanced. If you have ever seen your child come home on a high after eating sweets at a birthday party and then crash, you know what I'm talking about. As adults, I think we often become desensitized to those experiences in our own bodies, but they are still happening even if we have gotten used to them.

There is a system called the glycemic index (GI) used for ranking foods according to how quickly the body digests the carbohydrates in them. The GI can enhance your understanding of how your body experiences a sugar high. It's a useful tool, especially if you're concerned about your blood glucose levels, and it can be really eye opening to check the GI on some of the foods that you enjoy. I don't like to get too hung up on this number, because most foods you'll be eating more of on The Program have a naturally lower GI. You can also lower the GI impact of a particular food by eating it in combination with protein, fat, or fiber, which all tend to slow the digestive process, but The Program generally follows the principle that eating lower on the GI scale is better, and that definitely means reducing sugar.

The American Heart Association recommends that most men limit the amount of added sugar in their diet (not the kind that occurs naturally in fruit) to 9 teaspoons (36 grams) daily and that most women stop at 6 teaspoons (24 grams). If you track your sugar intake for a day or two before starting The Program, you're probably going to find that you are exceeding that recommendation. Keep in mind that there are about 30 different ways sugar can be listed on an ingredient label!

Honey or real maple syrup are better, less-processed alternatives when you use added sweeteners. I like to use raw manuka honey, which has active anti-inflammatory cultures. But this is all still sugar, so it should be used sparingly. There is really no need for refined sugar (white or brown) or liquid sugar on The Program or in your diet. If that is going to be a radical change for you, try not to be overwhelmed by it but consider making small changes in the right direction by reducing your sugar intake before you start The Program.

By the way, if a product that satisfies your sweet tooth is labeled "low sugar," "reduced sugar," "light," "calorie-free," or "no added sugar," it probably has chemically manufactured artificial sweeteners. These do not support your health. There are multiple types available and there is conflicting, confusing evidence about their safety and at what level of use they may interfere with healthy bacteria in your gut. I'm not a scientist, but here's what I know: these concentrated sweeteners, even if they turn out to be safe and help with weight loss or maintenance, are so intensely sweet that they distort your palate when you use them on a routine basis. When you eliminate them or use them less often, you will start to find naturally sweet things, like strawberries, more delicious and satisfying.

Stevia would be my choice if you are going to use an artificial sweetener at all. Stevia is plant-based, and I've included it as a possibility in a few of my recipes for people who want a bit of sweetness. But try to reduce your use of it, just as an experiment, and let your taste buds adjust. As a general rule, if you want to have something sweet to eat beyond a piece of fruit, I'd rather see you eat a little bit of sweetener in a relatively natural state combined with a protein source. A plain yogurt mixed with a little fruit or honey is a better choice than a chemically flavored, artificially sweetened, sugar-free, fat-free yogurt.

Fiber

Nonsoluble fiber is a kind of carbohydrate that our bodies can't digest that helps your digestive system function properly. This is the kind of fiber you find in fruits, seeds, and vegetable skins. Soluble fiber, the kind you find in oats and beans, has been shown to promote health and reduce the risk of heart disease and certain cancers. Most people don't get enough of either type and overlook fiber and the role it can play in weight loss and in overall health.

Remember when we talked about the problem with glucose and foods with a high GI? Fiber helps your body regulate that, by slowing down the rate at which sugar enters your bloodstream. Fiber also aids your digestion by promoting healthy bacteria in your gut, prevents constipation, and can help reduce your cholesterol. Finally, because it takes more time for your body to digest fiber, it keeps you feeling full, which will help you if you are adjusting to eating less.

Women should shoot to have 25 grams of fiber every day, and men should ideally have 38 grams per day. I don't want to give you a lot of numbers to track, but try looking at the fiber content of the foods you eat normally for a day or two. This is going to be the opposite of the sugar tracking: you'll probably be surprised at how little you get relative to the recommendations. See, I'm actually telling you to eat more of something!

HOW YOU EAT

In addition to paying attention to what kind of food you're using to fuel your body, you need to think about how much of it you eat. I don't know how tall you are, how old you are, how much you weigh, how much you want to weigh, or how active you are. These factors all play into how much you need to eat each day to function at your best.

Even if the food on your plate is very healthy, it is possible to have more than you need—and many of us have gotten confused about what full should feel like. Everything seems to have gotten bigger: our dishes are oversized, we eat prepared foods more often (either as prepared takeout or in a restaurant), and take advantage of super-sized food and beverage "deals" when we shop. Most of us can benefit from learning about reasonable portion sizes and how to feel satisfied by them.

I think the easiest way to get realistic about portions is to downsize your dinner plate to something that's between 7 and 9 inches across and fill it according to the PCF ratio you are following for that meal. That plate might have about half of it filled with nonstarchy vegetables, a quarter of it filled with lean protein, and a quarter of it with a complex carbohydrate. Many people find that using a smaller plate helps them control their portions without getting hung up on measurements or calories. If this system might work for you, make sure to fill your plate at the stove or in the kitchen, then bring that plate to the table, rather than serving the food family style.

If you still feel hungry when your plate is clean, give yourself at least 20 minutes to evaluate your hunger before you decide to have seconds. Drink a glass of water, get up from the table, or do something else in the meantime. Most people really feel okay when they check back in after giving their brains a chance to catch up to their stomach and register that feeling of being done. If you decide that you are truly hungry and are going to have more, you'll be making the choice in a conscious way.

To see if you are in tune with appropriate portion sizes, you can start educating yourself, as an exercise, by comparing the size of a serving on your favorite packaged food with how much you actually eat in a normal sitting. That is usually eye opening. An ordinary box of pasta from your supermarket shelf generally has eight servings in it, according to the label. Do you usually get eight meals out of one box? You can also look at what a recommended serving of something really is. The USDA counts 1 ounce of bread, grain, or cereal as a serving. The next time you buy a bagel, put it on the scale at your grocery store or ask your bagel guy to weigh it, just for kicks. If you are buying it in the United States, one bagel is probably between 5 and 8 ounces. Now, this kind of thing works the other way, too. For example, if I tell someone that they should really have eight servings of fruit and vegetables a day, they might say that they couldn't possibly eat that much. But if you understand that for most fruits and vegetables, a serving is about ½ cup, it seems much easier.

What Is a Serving?

GRAINS/STARCHES

1 slice bread
1 ounce ready-to-eat cereal
½ cup cooked cereal, rice, or pasta (about the size of half a baseball)

VEGETABLES

1 cup raw leafy vegetables
½ cup other vegetables
½ cup vegetable juice

FRUITS

1 small fruit
1 cup berries
½ cup juice

MEAT, POULTRY, FISH, DRY BEANS, AND NUTS

2–3 ounces cooked lean meat, poultry, or fish
½ cup cooked dry beans
2 tablespoons peanut butter

MILK, YOGURT, AND CHEESE

1 cup of fat-free or low-fat milk or yogurt
1½ ounces fat-free or low-fat cheese

The recommended serving sizes are a lot smaller than most people think. If you don't want to bother measuring things out precisely, there are visual ways to think about serving sizes. Whichever way you choose to monitor your portion sizes—through your small plate, by measuring, or by imagining an analogous item—you'll get the hang of it quickly and it will become instinctive. Many people are pretty surprised to realize how much they have been eating, so this may be an important reality check for you.

Serving Size Cues

3 ounces meat = deck of cards or computer mouse
3 ounces fish = checkbook
1 ounce cheese = 4 dice
1 medium fruit = baseball
1 cup of raw leafy greens = small fist
½ cup = tennis ball
¼ cup = golf ball
1 teaspoon = fingertip or one die
1 tablespoon = thumb tip

You aren't going to be eating much packaged food on The Program, but if and when you do, make sure you are paying attention to the serving size on the food label. Things like nuts or granola can often be surprisingly calorie-dense, even though they have many redeeming nutritional qualities and a legitimate place in a healthy diet. So I'm not asking you to count calories, but do tune into what a "serving" really is. Break out the measuring cups or spoons for a couple days to get the hang of it if you need to. It may surprise you. The good news is that getting a more instinctive sense of how much you really need will help you make food choices that are better fuel for your body.

You have more control over your food when you prepare it at home. I like the convenience of eating out or ordering in just like you probably do, but portions tend to be much larger than you need when they come from a restaurant and will usually have been prepared with larger quantities of oil or butter than you would use at home. Try to prepare your own food during your first cycle through The Program, so you can know exactly what you're taking in. You'll also be adjusting your expectations: when you've been eating clean, your palate will recognize the heavier ingredients in other foods and perhaps resist larger quantities of them, which will make your life that much easier as you keep making healthy choices.

One More Thing

I know I'm talking about food as a form of fuel and in terms of macro- and micronutrients, but I want you to know that I understand that food is one of life's pleasures, and it is one of mine. I love to eat. I care about food and how it tastes. I'm still evolving as a cook, but I enjoy creating breakfast smoothies and dinner scrambles, introducing my son to new foods, and sharing great meals with my friends and family. My Sunday rituals include going to my local farmer's market. When I travel, I enjoy connecting with people who are growing and making food they care about. I get that what we eat is both personal and social, and that it needs to taste good in addition to being good for us. The Program might change your diet, but it doesn't have to change the fact that food might be a source of pleasure and meaning in your life. I hope you find that what you enjoy eating and how you enjoy it gets even better.

Eating to Cleanse

Even though I'm calling these Cleanse days, please know that you are not dirty. I know the body has a very good system for cleaning and "detoxifying" itself. But we give our bodies a big job every day. Your liver, kidneys, colon, and other systems are removing toxins stored in your organs, tissues, and fat every day all by themselves. The way you're going to eat over the next few days is going to lighten their load a little bit and help prepare your body to maximize all the nutrient-rich food you're going to use to fuel yourself on The Program. The digestive system is very important for your overall health, and evidence suggests that gut health plays a role in weight loss as well. The recipes I provide for Cleanse days make use of ingredients that support your health in these key areas.

Everyone's experience is different, and I don't know how much of a change the Cleanse days will be from how you're already eating. Some of my clients report that after eating in the Cleanse style for a few days they experience improvement with bloating, indigestion, feelings of sluggishness, concentration, headaches, skin, and energy. Many of them experience weight loss. In other words, most of them feel better than they have been feeling. In addition to rebalancing your blood glucose and gut health, fighting inflammation in the body, and burning some fat, eating "clean" is also a good way to adjust your eating habits and practice a little discipline.

You are going to take a break from coffee, sugar, alcohol, and dairy as well as eliminate all processed food and animal protein over the next 4 days. Don't close the book! It's only 4 days. If you are very caffeine-dependent, you might try eliminating or reducing your coffee or tea intake for a couple of days before starting The Program, so that any effects of that withdrawal don't make the Cleanse days unpleasant for you. But some people choose to do it all cold turkey. It's up to you.

By the way, resist any temptation you might have to overeat the day before the cleanse. You want to reduce inflammation and bring your body back into balance, and you're just going to make it harder on yourself if you go crazy the night before. This is not a fad diet, and you're not permanently eliminating anything. And you may just have to trust me, but I think you're going to find that what you want to eat will change over time as you follow The Program. But for now, if you're feeling anxious about it, just remind yourself that this is only 4 days and take it one day—or even one meal—at a time.

You are not going to be hungry because this is not a fast. The smoothies and soups will give you vitamins and minerals from fresh, raw, whole vegetables, fruits, and nuts in a way that is easy for your body to digest and use. You will be able to exercise in the ways I suggest during the cleanse days. Remember, this is not a crash diet; it's about feeling better. Moving will help you do that.

For the first 4 days, you are going to drink three smoothies and eat three soups each day. You can eat them in any order you want; just space them through the day. You can make all your smoothies and soups using the recipes I provide or you can substitute your own, as long as you follow my basic rules. The smoothies and soups must all contain three of four essential elements that I describe below, and you need one vegetable-based soup and one bean-based soup. Otherwise, it's pretty flexible. You can choose which ones you want to make from the recipes I've provided for Cleanse days.

Smoothies

I love my morning smoothies and think they are an efficient, delicious way of starting the day. You're going to have three of them each day during the first four Cleanse days of The Program. You can make the same smoothie over and over again during those days if you like, or you can try all the recipes—it's up to you. I've offered "amped-up" versions of all the smoothies if you want to make them later in The Program when you need more fuel or if you're making them for people who aren't eating to cleanse. If you want to go off-menu and purchase or make a substitute smoothie, make sure it contains at least three of what I call the Core Four elements in each category. Also, this is not really about counting calories, but the Cleanse versions of the smoothies come in at around 200 calories per serving. If you're buying one, you need to keep that in mind. In most cases, I think you'll get more volume if you make one of the ones from my recipes. They're really easy!

CORE FOUR FOR SMOOTHIES

Whichever smoothies you choose, you'll find yourself trying three of the Core Four:

Fit Fats (Unsaturated Fats): Fat is your friend, at least the kinds I'm talking about. These include avocado, coconut, nuts, seeds, natural nut butters, and the healthy fat (omega-3s) found in chia and flaxseed, as well as fish such as salmon. Choosing these healthy fats, especially the omega-3 sources, will help to reduce inflammation in the body, fuel your cells, and keep your blood sugar in balance. These fats also help fight hunger if you are eating less than you're used to during the Cleanse days.

Polyphenols: Our bodies have molecules called free radicals that can cause a lot of damage, especially to the arteries. Polyphenols are compounds found in plants that help prevent that damage. There is some evidence that they act as antioxidants in the body and have potential health benefits, including reducing the risk of heart disease, preventing cancer, and boosting good microorganisms in your digestive system. Polyphenols are found in a variety of foods, including fruits and vegetables, spices (especially dried peppermint, cloves, and star anise), cocoa powder, dark chocolate, flaxseed meal, coffee, and green tea. Just-picked fruits and vegetables generally have higher levels of polyphenols compared with produce that's been sitting in your refrigerator for a while, so maybe that's a little motivation to buy as fresh as you can and use it sooner rather than later. Also, don't be too quick to peel: there is often a high concentration of polyphenols in the skin of your produce.

Leafy Greens: These are loaded with antioxidants, vitamins, and minerals. In addition to fighting inflammation, leafy greens are a good fiber source that will help you feel fuller on cleanse days while being super low in calories. Studies show that a little more than one serving of leafy greens daily can decrease your risk of diabetes by 14 percent! If you don't already love the taste of greens, many people find it easier to get their fill in a blended form, so try the green smoothies if that's you. There are differences in the ways that greens taste, too. If you don't like iceberg or romaine lettuce, try arugula, watercress, and butterhead. Try spinach, kale, Swiss chard, mustard greens, collards, cabbage, and broccoli. Try them raw and cooked and in combinations with other ingredients until you find some favorites.

Power Protein: Protein powder and yogurt and/or kefir are the main protein sources for smoothies. Different types of protein powder are interchangeable in the recipes, but give whey-based proteins a try if you tolerate dairy, especially if you're drinking one after a Build workout. Whey protein is generally easily digested and stimulates muscle growth well. Seventy percent of the immune system is in your gut. Yogurt and kefir contain probiotics that are important for gut health and help with your immune function, so those are also good choices that you can use as your primary form of protein in the smoothies if you prefer. Emerging research also suggests an association between gut bacteria and weight, so the dairy-based options offer this benefit as well. If you don't tolerate dairy, pea- and hemp-based protein powders are also solid protein options. You can also blend powders to ensure that all of the amino acids are provided to make a "complete" protein. There are many soy-based protein powders on the market, and while you can use them in the smoothies, these aren't my preference because of emerging and conflicting evidence about the effects overconsumption of soy may have in certain populations. Whey-, pea-, and hemp-based powders don't seem to be raising the same concerns, so I'd encourage you to give them a try first if you are new to protein powders.

Soups

You'll be eating three soups a day during the Cleanse days, and you'll want to make at least one vegetable-based and one bean-based option. Of course, you can make all of them, either for use during the Cleanse or freeze them to eat at any other point in The Program. You'll see suggestions for increasing their nutritional content or pairing them with other foods in the recipe section if you're cooking for family members who are not also eating to cleanse.

It's fine to create your own soup or buy premade options, but they must contain three out of four of the Core Four options for soup. Bean-based soups should contain approximately 200 calories per serving, and vegetable soups should contain approximately 100 calories per serving. I think the recipes provided are very satisfying relative to the calorie count; other options in your grocery store may be less so. Keep an eye on the serving size of anything you buy, and if the caloric equivalent seems small, try making one of mine.

CORE FOUR FOR SOUP

Whichever soups you choose to make, you're going to be using a combination of the following core elements, which I hope you'll keep incorporating into your diet throughout The Program.

Spices/Herbs: Many are polyphenols and contain bioactive compounds that some evidence suggests may help to reduce inflammation in the body. Sage, thyme, ginger, rosemary, marjoram, and oregano have all been used for centuries as folk medicine, as have chile pepper, black pepper, and cinnamon. But they also taste great and give your soups flavor and depth without added fat or calories. The soup recipes for The Program were developed to take advantage of these properties.

Cruciferous Vegetables: It is so worth developing a taste for these good guys— kale, sprouts, cauliflower, cabbage, bok choy, broccoli, arugula—if you haven't already. These are loaded with antioxidants, vitamins, and minerals and are great fiber sources, which will help you feel fuller on cleanse days. Some people find soups an easier way to incorporate these ingredients in their diet rather than raw or steamed. You should try to eat some one way or another every day, and most of the soups will cover this one for you.

Allium Family: These include onions, garlic, shallots, scallions, and leeks, which people have used for years for their health benefits. Research tells us that they contain organosulfides, a type of polyphenol that is believed to have antioxidant properties. This is great news because these plants can provide a really rich, pungent flavor base for your soups (and many other meals) without added calories and fat. Onions have a higher polyphenol and flavonoid content than other members of the allium group, but you'll benefit from all of them.

Beans: Kidney beans, black beans, chickpeas, lentils—you name it, they're all good! You can use mine or pick a recipe that has other types of beans you like. Beans are an excellent source of plant-based protein and fiber, which will help keep you full, and they also contain antioxidants to help fight inflammation. They are generally a quality source of magnesium, which most people don't get enough of. Beans are also a slowly digested carbohydrate which helps keep blood sugar in check. The fact that beans make satisfying and delicious meals is almost a bonus.

You'll want to eat one serving of a bean-based soup and two servings of a vegetable soup each day during the Cleanse.

The smoothies and soups can be eaten in any order. I'd space them out every 2–3 hours. Here are different ways your first Cleanse day might look:

Option 1	Option 2	Option 3 Choose Your Own
Java Mocha Smoothie	Green Tea Smoothie	Smoothie (Core 3)
Chocolate-Covered Strawberry Smoothie	Cherry Almond Smoothie	Smoothie (Core 3)
Carrot-Ginger Soup	Tomato-Cucumber Gazpacho	Vegetable-based soup
Blueberry Pear Smoothie	Tropical Kale Smoothie	Smoothie (Core 3)
White Bean and Tuscan Kale Soup	Black Bean Soup with Pico de Gallo	Bean-based soup
Carrot-Ginger Soup	Tomato-Cucumber Gazpacho	Vegetable-based soup

A couple of notes about Cleanse days:

- *If you need to lose more than 50 pounds, are younger than 30, a woman who is taller than 5'8", or a man who is taller than 6', you can make one additional smoothie on Cleanse days and drink it at any point during the day.*
- If you are hungry between soups and smoothies, snack on vegetable broth or raw nonstarchy vegetables in any quantity. Some people find particular raw vegetables difficult to digest, and part of the point of the Cleanse days is to let your digestive system take it easy, but if you're hungry or missing the "crunch" from your food during these days, feel free to snack on nonstarchy vegetables that work for you.
- All of the soup and smoothie recipes contain tips to increase calories and/or add protein so that you can incorporate them into your menu plan again during The Program if you like them and want to make them even more substantial, depending on your workout.

BURN AND BUILD

After the first 4 days of The Program, you'll start to ramp up your workouts and you'll need to increase and adjust what you eat, according to the type of workout I have you doing each day. The days have some things in common. On both days, you'll eat at least:

Six servings of vegetables and fruit
One to two servings of dairy
Protein and fat at every meal

On Build days, you'll be shooting for a PCF ratio of 30/40/30. That means that your food over the course of the day should be made up of about 30 percent protein, 40 percent complex carbohydrates, and 30 percent fat. Don't worry, you aren't going to need to calculate any of that. If you follow the meal plan, I've done it all for you, or given you the equivalent values so you can substitute things without going off track if you don't find my suggestions appealing. You'll notice that one of your meals will not contain any grain or starch, but that meal can have more protein and vegetables. You also have protein-oriented snacks that are optimal on these days.

An optimal Build day might look like this:

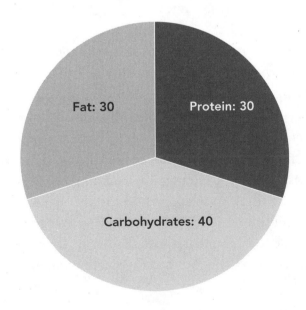

On Burn days, you are going to eat toward a daily PCF ratio of 25/50/25. That means that your food over the course of the days you are doing Burn workouts should be made up of about 25 percent protein, 50 percent complex carbohydrates, and 25 percent fat. You'll notice you can have more grain and/or fruit servings during these days.

An optimal Burn day might look like this:

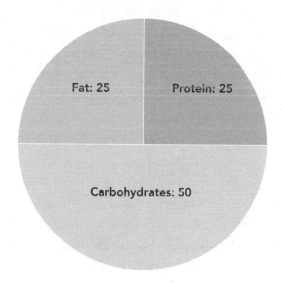

When you look at all the meal plans, you'll notice that while the PCF ratios for Burn and Build days are consistent, the food exchanges vary according to the sample menu. In other words, there are a lot of different ways to get to the correct balance of macronutrients in your day. The meal plans mix it up to keep it interesting. So make sure that if you substitute meals or snacks by using the exchanges, you actually use the ones for that particular meal or day.

Eating this way should not be a chore, and once you get used to it, it's pretty simple. You don't have to count calories or grams of anything. I have provided calorie counts in the sample meal plans, though, for those of you who do like to keep track of them, and so that you can understand how much you are eating. If you feel you need to eat more, depending on your meals and goals, you can adjust your portion sizes, either during your first cycle of The Program or at any point in the future.

Notice that on both Burn and Build days you'll be eating protein with every meal (2–3 ounces at breakfast and 3–5 ounces at lunch and dinner). That's really important, both for feeling full and to protect and feed your muscle mass when you're working out. On Build days, you'll want to have your protein-packed snack after your Build workout, preferably within 30 minutes.

If you need to lose more than 50 pounds, are younger than 30, a woman who is taller than 5'8', or a man over 6' tall, you can eat an extra snack every day from the appropriate list and can feel free to add an additional ounce or two of protein per meal. I've designed two 20-minute workouts for each day, which you will read about in the Sweat section of The Program, but if you choose to do additional exercise on any day so that your total amount of time spent working out is 90 minutes or more, you should also have an additional snack regardless of your size.

RELAX DAY RULES

On the last day of the first cycle of The Program, I introduce what I'm calling a Relax eating day. The reality is that food is not only fuel, it is a source of pleasure, a part of your heritage, and a way of celebrating and connecting with people you care about. Any realistic eating plan has to make room for that in your life. The key is not to let that relaxing derail your motivation to keep eating well most of the time or to undo any progress you made by being disciplined about your eating and workouts. I see clients struggle with both of those challenges. Here's my best advice. Choose what kind of workout you want to do on your Relax day: it can be one of my Burn or Build workouts that you particularly enjoyed, or it can be something else that you love to do or want to try. You can go for a hike, bike ride, or run; go kayaking; ice skate; play tennis or basketball—anything you might look forward to but not have time to explore during a normal day. I know your life is busy, and the regular workouts on The Program are designed to be about 20 minutes of maximum effort to fit into a crowded schedule. I'm imagining a Relax day to be one where you may have a bit more time and space to try other ways of moving that inspire you.

Choose your basic eating plan for your Relax day based on your workout (Is it more of a Burn or a Build? How long will you do it for?) and eat on plan for the majority of the day, but, if you want to, add a reasonable treat to your menu. For me, that might be a burger and a beer, both things I love but wouldn't eat on a daily basis. I don't know what you'll want; it could be a glass of wine, a dessert, a pasta dish, bread made with white flour. Whatever it is, be intentional about it. Make it something you really want, and keep your portions reasonable. Be clear with yourself: the calories from alcohol or chocolate cake are not offering you nutritious fuel. They are satisfying another function, one that should have a place in your life that stays in check if you want to stay healthy.

Now, what if you go a little crazy and relax your eating plan beyond your intentions? This happens, and it's a bit of a live and learn situation. Notice if there is a pattern to the types of foods or situations that challenge your discipline, and keep it in mind. The most important thing is committing back to The Program. For some of my clients, that might mean repeating a Cleanse Day, in whole or in part. You do not have to do this; you can just rotate right back into a Burn or Build schedule of eating that makes sense for you. But if you feel your motivation waning in the wake of a Relax meal or day, take action and head back to the Cleanse menus. For example, if you had a piece of cake on your Relax day, maybe you want to replace one meal tomorrow with one of the Cleanse smoothies. If you had a glass of wine with that piece of cake, maybe you want to swap out two meals from your next day with a Cleanse smoothie or soup. If you have three or more "treats" during your Relax day, consider following up with a full Cleanse day from the beginning of The Program.

What Counts as a Treat:

Alcohol
Extra starch serving (pasta, bread, chips, etc.)
Refined grains
Dessert or sweets
Foods containing high amounts of fat (fried food, cheese, etc.)

PAYING ATTENTION

Most of us eat too quickly and don't pay much attention to our food. It takes about 20 minutes for the brain to register that our stomachs are full, so when we eat quickly and mindlessly, it's easy to overeat before we get that message. We also don't tend to really appreciate or enjoy what we're eating when we're distracted. So, turn off your TV, put your phone in its charger, and try to really pay attention to your next meal.

Use the meal plans for the next 21 days to reset your appetite, your palate, and your body. I've given you the food exchanges and calorie counts for each meal to make it as easy as possible for you to switch ingredients or meals for things that are appealing to you. These numbers are approximate and rounded, they are meant to give you general guidance and ease your ability to stay on track with the Program when you want to eat differently. But I hope you'll challenge yourself to try some new things during this time as well, and experiment with ways of incorporating healthy food into your diet. Don't give up on anything right away, especially if it's in one of the Core Four families! Try other strategies. For example, if you don't like kale raw in a salad, try blending it in a smoothie, or cooking it in a little bit of one of the fit fats with a spice that appeals to you. The menu plans that follow are just an example. You will use them as building blocks to eat well forever, and that means it all needs to taste good to you!

DAY BY DAY

DAY 1: CLEANSE

Cleanse Day 1		1,019 calories
Java Mocha Smoothie	1 dairy, ½ fruit, 1 fat	192
Carrot-Ginger Soup	3 vegetables, ½ fat	128
Green Tea Smoothie	3 protein, 1 fruit, ½ vegetable, 1 fat	200
Blueberry Pear Smoothie	1 dairy, 1 fruit, ½ vegetable, 1 fat	211
White Bean and Tuscan Kale Soup	1 starch, 2+ vegetables, ½ fat, 1 protein	160
Carrot-Ginger Soup	3 vegetables, ½ fat	128
Fitness assessment		
Slow-burn cardio		

DAY 2: CLEANSE

Cleanse Day 2		1,014 calories
Green Tea Smoothie	3 protein, 1 fruit, ½ vegetable, 1 fat	200
Cherry Almond Smoothie	3 protein, 2 fruits, 1 vegetable, 2 fats	216
Tomato-Cucumber Gazpacho	2 vegetables, 1 fat	92
Chocolate-Covered Strawberry Smoothie	3 protein, 1 fruit, 1 fat	214
White Bean and Tuscan Kale Soup	1 starch, 2+ vegetables, ½ fat, 1 protein	160
Carrot-Ginger Soup	3 vegetables, ½ fat	128
Fitness assessment		
Slow-burn cardio		

DAY 3: CLEANSE

Cleanse Day 3		1,030 calories
Blueberry Pear Smoothie	1 dairy, 1 fruit, ½ vegetable, 1 fat	211
Java Mocha Smoothie	1 dairy, ½ fruit, 1 fat	192
Curried Cauliflower Soup	2 vegetables, 1 fat	103
Tropical Kale Smoothie	1 dairy, 1 fruit, ½ vegetable, 1 fat	217
Black Bean Soup with Pico de Gallo	1½ starch, 2 vegetables, ½ fat, 2 proteins	220
Mushroom and Bok Choy Soup	3 vegetables, ½ fat	104
Fitness assessment		
Slow-burn cardio		

DAY 4: CLEANSE

Cleanse Day 4		957 calories
Cherry Almond Smoothie	3 protein, 1 fruit, ½ vegetable, 1 fat	220
Chocolate-Covered Strawberry Smoothie	3 protein, 1 fruit, 1 fat	214
Green Tea Smoothie	3 protein, 1 fruit, ½ vegetable, 1 fat	200
Black Bean Soup with Pico de Gallo	1½ starch, 2 vegetables, ½ fat, 2 proteins	220
Curried Cauliflower Soup	2 vegetables, 1 fat	103
Fitness assessment		
Slow-burn cardio		

DAY 5: BURN

Burn Day 5	PCF ratio 25/50/25	1,220 calories
Wake-up Workout		
B: Upgraded Green Tea Smoothie	3 protein, 2 fruits, ½ vegetable, 2 fats	290
L: Mexican Scramble Soft Taco + ½ mango	1½ starches, 4 protein, 1 fruit, 1 vegetable, 2 fats	410
S: 6 ounces plain or vanilla fat-free Greek yogurt with ½ cup berries	1 dairy, ½ fruit, 1 fat	180
D: Shrimp Stir-Fry	2 starches, 3 protein, 2 vegetables, 2 fats	340
Burn workout		

Exchanges for day: 3½ starches, 1 dairy, 10 protein, 3½ fruits, 3½ vegetables, 7 fats

DAY 6: BUILD

Build Day 6	PCF ratio 30/40/30	1,270 calories
Wake-up Workout		
B: Power Protein Pancakes	1½ starch, ½ dairy, 2½ protein, ½ fruit	340
L: Quinoa Chicken Salad + 1 small peach	1½ starch, 4 protein, 1 fruit, 2 vegetables, 1 fat	410
S: 1 (1 ounce) low-fat string cheese and 1 (100-calorie) pack of almonds	1 dairy, 1 fat	160
D: Turkey Taco Wraps and Salad	4 protein, 4 vegetables, 2 fats	360
Build workout		

Exchanges for day: 3 starches, 1½ dairy, 10½ protein, 1½ fruits, 6 vegetables, 4 fats

DAY 7: BURN

Burn Day 7	PCF ratio 25/50/25	1,330 calories
Wake-up Workout		
B: Oatmeal Chia Porridge	1½ starch, 1 dairy, 3 protein, ½ fruit, 1 fat	410
L: California Turkey Wrap + 1 cup carrots + 1 cup honeydew melon	1½ starches, 3 protein, 1 fruit, 2 vegetables, 1 fat, 1+ dairy	450
S: 2 small kiwis and 7 walnut halves	1 fruit, 1 fat	180
D: Baked Pork Chop with Roasted Sweet Potato and Brussels Sprouts	1½ starches, 3 protein, 1½ vegetables, 1 fat	290
Burn workout		

Exchanges for day: 4½ starches, 2+ dairy, 9 protein, 2½ fruits, 3½ vegetables, 4 fats

DAY 8: BUILD

Build Day 8	PCF ratio 30/40/30	1,250 calories
Wake-up Workout		
B: Pumpkin Smoothie	1 dairy, 3 protein, 1 fruit, 1 fat	340
L: Tuna Spinach Salad + 1 small pear	1 starch, 4 protein, 1 fruit, 1½ vegetables, 1 fat	390
S: ½ cup steamed edamame	2 protein	120
D: Fajita Salad	1 starch, 4 protein, 3½ vegetables, 1 fat	400
Build workout		

Exchanges for day: 2 starches, 1 dairy, 13 protein, 2 fruits, 5 vegetables, 3 fats

DAY 9: BURN

Burn Day 9	PCF ratio 25/50/25	1,220 calories
Wake-up Workout		
B: Oatmeal Breakfast Cookies	1½ starches, 1 protein, 1 fruit, 2 fats	310
L: Chicken Caesar Wrap + ½ cup carrots + 1 small orange	1½ starches, 3 protein, 1 fruit, 1½ vegetables, 1 fat	420
S: 6 ounces plain fat-free Greek yogurt with ½ cup berries and stevia	1 dairy, 1 fruit	140
D: Sweet and Spicy Chicken Breast with Mashed Sweet Potatoes and Broccoli	1½ starch, 3 protein, 1½ vegetables, 1 fat	350
Burn workout		

Exchanges for day: 1½ starches, 1 dairy, 7 protein, 3 fruit, 4 vegetables, 4 fats

DAY 10: BUILD

Build Day 10	PCF ratio 30/40/30	1,285 calories
Wake-up Workout		
B: Upgraded Java Mocha Smoothie	1+ dairy, 2 fruits, 2 fats	310
L: Turkey Mushroom Scramble + ½ English muffin	1 starch, 4 protein, 1½ vegetables, 2 fats	330
S: 2 ounces lean jerky (turkey or bison) and one medium apple	2 protein, 1 fruit	255
D: Salmon, Roasted Beet, and Goat Cheese Salad for Two plus one whole grain roll	1 starch, 4 protein, ½ dairy, 2 vegetables, 1 fat	390
Build workout		

Exchanges for day: 2 starches; 1½+ dairy, 10 protein, 3 fruits, 3½ vegetables, 5 fats

DAY 11: BURN

Burn Day 11	PCF ratio 25/50/25	1,210 calories
Wake-up Workout		
B: Upgraded Blueberry Pear Smoothie	1 dairy, 1½ protein, 2 fruits, 1 vegetable, 1 fat	320
L: Chicken Caprese Wrap + 1 cup grapes	1½ starches, 2 protein, 1 dairy, 1 fruit, 2 vegetables	390
S: 1 small banana + 1 tablespoon natural peanut butter	1 fruit, 1 fat	200
D: Shrimp Sautéed with Broccoli + Rice	1½ starches, 4 protein, 1½ vegetables, 1 fat, ½ dairy	300
Burn workout		

Exchanges for day: 3 starches, 2½ dairy, 7½ protein, 4 fruits, 4½ vegetables, 3 fats

DAY 12: BUILD

Build Day 12	PCF ratio 30/40/30	1,225 calories
Wake-up Workout		
B: Baked Egg "Muffins" + 1 small orange	½ dairy, 2½ protein, 1 fruit, ¼ vegetable	260
L: Buffalo Chicken Salad + 1 cup strawberries	1½ starch, ½ dairy, 4 protein, 1 fruit, 1½ vegetables, 1 fat	420
S: 6 ounces plain or vanilla fat-free Greek yogurt with 2 tablespoons sunflower seeds	1 dairy, 2 fats	190
D: Turkey Meatballs and Marinara with Zucchini Noodles	1 starch, 4 protein, 4 vegetables, 1 fat	355
Build workout		

Exchanges for day: 2½ starches, 2 dairy, 10½ protein, 2 fruits, 5¾ vegetables, 4 fats

DAY 13: BURN

Burn Day 13	PCF ratio 25/50/25	1,325 calories
Wake-up Workout		
B: Peanut Butter/Berry/Egg White Oatmeal	2 starches, 1½ protein, 1 fruit, 2 fats	350
L: Turkey Wrap with Veggies + 1 small apple	1½ starches, 1+ dairy, 2 protein, 1 fruit, 3 vegetables	420
S: 1 small orange + 1 hard-boiled egg	1 protein, 1 fruit	130
D: 3 ounces flank steak + 1 cup beets + ½ cup green beans	3 protein, 1½ vegetables, 2 fat	425
Burn workout		

Exchanges for day: 3½ starches, 1+ dairy, 4½ protein, 3 fruits, 6 vegetables, 4 fats

DAY 14: BUILD

Build Day 14	PCF ratio 30/40/30	1,310 calories
Wake-up Workout		
B: Avocado Egg White Bake	2 protein, 1 fruit, 2+ fats	290
L: Chicken Bean Lettuce Wraps	1 starch, 4 protein, 1 fruit, 3 vegetables, 1 fat	420
S: 2 ounces lean jerky (turkey or bison)	2 protein	160
D: Salmon Cakes with Dill Sauce and Roasted Asparagus	1 starch, 1 dairy, 4 protein, 3 vegetables, 1 fat	440
Build workout		

Exchanges for day: 2 starches, 1 dairy, 12 protein, 2 fruits, 6 vegetables, 4+ fats

DAY 15: BURN

Burn Day 15	PCF ratio 25/50/25	1,320 calories
Wake-up Workout		
B: 1 piece whole wheat toast topped with 1 tablespoon peanut butter + ½ cup blueberries + 1 whole egg plus 1 egg white, hard-boiled	1 starch, 1 fruit, 2 protein, 1 fat	390
L: Chicken, Bean, Rice, and Avocado Bowl + 2 kiwis	2 starches, 4 protein, 1 fruit, 1 vegetables, 1 fat	430
S: 6 ounces plain or vanilla fat-free Greek yogurt with ½ cup berries	1 dairy, 1 fruit	130
D: 3 ounces salmon + ⅓ cup quinoa + 1½ cups asparagus	1 starch, 3½ protein, 3 vegetables, 1 fat	370
Burn workout		

Exchanges for day: 4 starches, 1 dairy, 9½ protein, 3 fruits, 4 vegetables, 3 fats

DAY 16: BUILD

Build Day 16	PCF ratio 30/40/30	1,270 calories
Wake-up Workout		
B: Blueberry Chia Power Protein Pudding	1 dairy, 3 protein, ½ fruit, 2 fats	370
L: Salmon Salad Lettuce Wraps + 1 cup grapes	1 starch, 3 protein, 1 fruit, 1½ vegetables, 1 fat, ⅓ dairy	350
S: ½ cup low-fat cottage cheese and 1 cup raw cherry tomatoes	1 dairy, 1 vegetable	140
D: Chicken Salad with Quinoa, Cucumber, and Strawberries	1½ starch, 4 protein, 1 fruit, 2½ vegetables, 1 fat	410
Build workout		

Exchanges for day: 2½ starches, 1⅓ dairy, 10 protein, 2½ fruits, 5 vegetables, 4 fats

DAY 17: BURN

Burn Day 17	PCF ratio 25/50/25	1,365 calories
Wake-up Workout		
B: Breakfast Burrito + 1 cup sliced strawberries	1½ starches, 2 protein, 1 fruit, ½ dairy, 1 vegetables, 1 fat	395
L: Tortilla Pizza with Green Salad	1½ starches, 2 protein, 1 dairy, 3 vegetables, 1 fat	360
S: Small pear + 1 ounce low-fat string cheese	1 dairy, 1 fruit	160
D: Chicken and Vegetable Kabobs with Tzatziki + Rice	1 starch, 1 dairy, 3 protein, 2 vegetables, 2 fats	450
Burn workout		

Exchanges for day: 4 starches, 2½ dairy, 7 protein, 1 fruits, 6 vegetables, 4 fats

DAY 18: BUILD

Build Day 18	PCF ratio 30/40/30	1,205 calories
Wake-up Workout		
B: 1 slice whole wheat toast with ¾ cup cottage cheese, 1 cup chopped tomatoes 1 teaspoon butter (for toast, if desired) + ½ grapefruit	1 starch, 3 protein, 1 fruit, 1 vegetable, 1 fat	330
L: Greek Chicken Salad	3 protein, 1 dairy, 1 fruit, 2 vegetables, 1 fat	330
S: 6 ounces plain or vanilla fat-free Greek yogurt with 1 tablespoon sunflower seeds	1 dairy, 1 fat	140
D: 4 ounces grilled beef tenderloin with 1 cup sautéed green beans (in 1 teaspoon olive oil), ½ a baked sweet potato and 1 teaspoon butter (if desired)	1 starch, 4 protein, 3 vegetables, 2 fat	405
Build		

Exchanges for day: 2 starches, 2 dairy, 10 protein, 2 fruits, 6 vegetables, 5 fats

THE PROGRAM-DAY 19-BURN

Burn Day 19	PCF ratio 20/50/30	1,200 calories
Wake-up Workout		
B: Upgraded Tropical Kale Smoothie	1+ dairy, 2 fruits, 1½ vegetables, 1 fat	290
L: Greek Chicken and Veggie Pita Pocket + 2 clementines + 1 cup sliced cucumbers	1 starch, 3 protein, 1 fruit, 1½ vegetables, 1 fat	340
S: 1 small banana + 1 tablespoon natural peanut butter	1 fruit, 1 fat	180
D: Chicken Veggie Pasta	1½ starches, 3 protein, 1½ vegetables, 1 fat	390
Burn workout		

Exchanges for day: 2½ starches, 1+ dairy, 6 protein, 4 fruits, 4½ vegetables, 4 fats

DAY 20: BUILD

Build Day 20	PCF ratio 30/40/30	1,290 calories
Wake-up Workout		
B: Ham and Veggie Scramble and Toast + 1 cup honeydew melon	1 starch, 3 protein, ½ dairy, 1 fruit, 2 vegetables, ½ fat	370
L: Chicken "Tacos" + 1 cup sliced strawberries	4 protein, 1 fruit, ½ vegetables, 2 fats	310
S: 6 ounces plain or vanilla fat-free Greek yogurt with 2 tablespoons chia seeds	1 dairy, 2 fats	200
D: Portobello Beef Burger and Zucchini Fries with Marinara Sauce	1 starch, 4½ protein, 4 vegetables, 1 fat	410
Build workout		

Exchanges for day: 2 starches, 1½ dairy, 11½ protein, 2 fruits, 5½ vegetables, 5½ fats

DAY 21: BURN

Burn Day 21	PCF ratio 25/50/25	1,290 calories
Wake-up Workout		
B: Nut and Berry Cereal Parfait + Hard-Boiled Eggs	1 starch, 1+ dairy, 1½ protein, ½ fruit, 1 fat	370
L: Turkey Burger and Green Salad + 2 kiwis	1½ starches, 3 protein, 1 fruit, 2 vegetables, 2 fats	460
S: 1 cup grapes + 1 reduced-fat string cheese	1 dairy, 1 fruit	130
D: Chicken Fajitas	1½ starches, 3 protein, 2½ vegetables, 1 fat	330
Burn workout		

Exchanges for day: 4 starches, 2+ dairy, 7½ protein, 2½ fruits, 4½ vegetables, 4 fats

DAY 22: RELAX

We all have foods or drinks we enjoy that we know need to have a limited role in a healthy diet. Any plan has to make room for them if you're going to stick to it over the long haul. Now, we all crave different things, so I'm not sure what your relax day might look like. But I can show you one of mine so you can get a sense of what relax means…enjoy, but don't go crazy! It's really easy to undo a week's worth of self-discipline about eating and exercise. That's why I wait so long in The Program to suggest a Relax day: I'm hoping, at this point, that you'll be satisfied with relatively modest indulgence. This is an optional day at this point in The Program. I don't know what's going on in your life or what your goals are, but you can use the last 21 days as a guide to help you keep moving toward them. But I know there are going to be days when you want to celebrate, take it easy, and enjoy. This is what that might look like.

Jessie's RELAX Day 22		
Wake-Up Workout		
B: Green Drink, Greek Yogurt, Berries	Cucumber, kale, avocado, lemon, lime, cayenne, apple cider vinegar	
L: Green Eggs Scramble	Eggs, turkey, bell pepper, avocado, tomatillo, cayenne	
S: Chicken Tacos (the chicken is the taco shell!)	Grilled chicken, avocado, bean sprouts, vegan mayo, cayenne, Greek pepperoncini	
D: Burger, Beer, Salad		
Weekend Challenge Workout and/or a hike		

Sweat

The quality of your food and how much of it you eat are critical components of your health. But you can be at a healthy weight and follow a "perfect" diet and still not be physically fit. As human beings, we were all designed to move, and if there is a better way to improve your overall quality of life than moving more, I don't know what it is. Most of us live from the neck up, but exercise allows us to live through our whole bodies. When I don't work out regularly, I miss it. If that is not a feeling you can identify with, I'm wondering if you have fully committed to exercise in the past. You may not like the gym—and that's fine—but if you stick with a workout routine and find a type of exercise that turns you on, it really changes you. Everyone I have ever worked with has gotten the exercise bug eventually. You have to keep at it long enough and keep trying different things to find what you like, but it's worth it. By the time you're done with The Program, a daily sweat will be as routine for you as eating and sleeping. Believe it or not, you're going to look forward to it and feel great.

THE WHY OF EXERCISE

Even if you haven't yet experienced how good exercise can feel, you know it's good for you. Being disciplined means doing things we know are important or good for us even when we don't want to do them. But if you're still at the stage where you find working out awkward or challenging, I think it helps you stay disciplined if you know why exercise is so good for you and can connect that knowledge to your personal motivation. So, if working out isn't already fun for you (and it will be, if you give it a little time), know that regular physical activity will directly improve your well-being in surprising ways.

Exercise improves your physical health

Different types of regular exercise can make you stronger and faster, improve your flexibility and agility, and make your body more efficient and functional. People who exercise regularly have better heart health, blood pressure, and cholesterol levels; have fewer neurologic and memory-related problems; are less likely to have cancer; and live longer compared with people who don't move a lot. You don't have to sweat hard to benefit from exercise: just 30 minutes of moderate activity (like brisk walking) each day is associated with a lower risk of diabetes, heart disease, and certain types of cancer. But there are benefits to pushing further for strength: most adults begin to lose skeletal muscle mass at a rate of up to 1 percent annually after age 25. Weight training can curtail that loss, strengthen your bones, and keep you stronger and less injury-prone for longer. Everyone can benefit from moving more and challenging themselves, but if you have been completely inactive, there is great news: you have the most to gain from starting a regular exercise program. It's not too late!

Exercise will help you get to and maintain a healthy weight

Regular exercise is not a free pass for a poor diet. What and how much you eat is a huge component of how much you weigh. But burning calories during exercise does allow you to eat a little more without gaining weight, and it will absolutely help you lose weight when you control your diet while you exercise.

There is nothing like the feeling of a great sweat after a long, hard workout, and one of the cool things you get, especially if you push at the end of a session, is something called an afterburn, which means that your metabolism is working harder for a bit after you're done exercising. If your exercise periods are broken up into smaller sessions throughout the day, you'll be boosting your metabolism more often and getting that afterburn multiple times, so that is one advantage to incorporating activity throughout your day. The Program workouts are designed with this in mind.

People who want to lose weight often focus on the cardio forms of working out, but strength training to help build and maintain lean muscle mass is critical because muscle burns more calories than fat, which raises your metabolism and helps you burn more when you're not exercising. Regular exercise is also hugely important in preventing weight gain and maintaining weight loss. The clients I've worked with who have lost extreme amounts of weight do best back in the "real world" when they stay active.

You will feed your mind

Regular aerobic exercise increases the flow of blood and oxygen to your brain, and stimulates chemicals in your brain that positively affect the health of your brain cells.

The evidence here is specifically for aerobic exercise, and it suggests that regular moderate activity can protect your cognitive functioning, regenerate nerve functioning in your brain, and improve your verbal memory and your ability to process information. I'm just going to go ahead and say that it seems like exercise makes you smarter.

Exercise will reduce feelings of stress

There is evidence that exercise can be as effective as therapy and meditation in helping people cope with stress. While it's natural for all of us to have moments of stress, many of us don't take it seriously as a physical health issue. Stress can increase bodily inflammation, lower immunity, raise your blood pressure, and generally makes you feel anxious and bad. I don't know of a better, cheaper, more natural stress reliever than the endorphins produced by exercise. Exercise won't just improve your mood; it will provide physiological benefits that improve your overall management of stress when you feel it. It should also help you sleep well at night, and being properly rested always makes things more manageable. When you are exhausted and out of breath at the end of a workout in which you put it all on the line, you are going to feel amazing. That's a serious reward to me, as much as any weight loss or improved body fat percentage.

Exercise helps you connect

Exercise doesn't just help you live longer, it helps you live better. Studies tell us that being active when you are older generally means you can be more independent, and people of all ages who are active usually have a greater sense of well-being than sedentary people. Physical activity is also a great way to meet other people. If you can find other people who like to train doing the same activities that you like to do, it is likely to be a source of friendship, support, and inclusion, not to mention a great motivator for you to keep moving! When you exercise out of doors, it will also support your sense of connection to nature, which will support your mental well-being—I know it helps mine!

You are going to have so much fun

You don't have to be "good" at an exercise to enjoy it. You do have to be game to get outside of your comfort zone and try enough different ones so that you can discover what you like. But I've yet to have a client who didn't eventually find something they felt good about doing. That's important, because if it's not fun, you won't stick with an exercise program, no two ways about it.

Look, it's painful to push yourself, and I don't know anyone who enjoys every minute of every workout, even though most people truly feel great afterward. But you do need to find ways to move that you enjoy. Be patient. Don't be afraid to try a lot of different things, and try not to be self-conscious about your skill level. It may take you a while to find what you truly love. Plus, most people do well with a varied mix of workouts so they don't get bored. Finally, give each activity a few tries before you give up on it, or even return to it later as your fitness level changes. I've had clients who preferred walking or hiking to running, then evolved into runners after several years. I've also had clients who were committed cyclists who started swimming in the winter when it was too cold to bike, and that became their primary form of cardio exercise even in peak cycling season. Someone I've worked with put on a pair of ice skates with her son last winter for the first time in 15 years and is still skating once a week on her own. You just never know what is going to energize you. Sometimes what your body is looking for at a given moment will surprise you. Be open to it. Anything that keeps you active is positive.

HAVE I SOLD YOU? LET'S GET STARTED

There is no magical secret. When you train properly, your body gets stronger, faster, and better. There are also no shortcuts. If you train correctly, you'll see improvements quickly, but if you hit it too hard and exercise to the point of exhaustion, you'll get burned out or, worse, injured. So you want workouts that challenge you, but at an appropriate pace for the long haul. That is different for everyone, and you'll spend some time during the first 4 days of The Program assessing your fitness level so you can find the right level workout for you. You also want balance in your training plan. The benefits of working out come from different forms of exercise. Everyone should want to strengthen muscles, avoid disease and injury, and improve cardiovascular health. Most of you probably also want to lose fat. These are related but different goals, and they are best achieved by a mix of movements. At each level of The Program, you'll be engaging in four different types of exercises to help you reach your goals efficiently.

The First 4 Days

During most of The Program, you're going to be following a movement program that alternates the focus of your workouts between Burn days and Build days. But the plan is designed to improve five key components of your physical fitness.

During the next 21 days you will be training in a strategic way designed to increase your strength, metabolic conditioning, athleticism, cardio endurance, and flexibility. You will be focusing on one or more of these five fitness elements at each workout.

BENEFITS OF STRENGTH TRAINING (BUILD)

Strength training protects bone health and muscle mass. As we age we lose muscle mass (some estimates indicate we lose between 5 and 7 pounds of muscle each decade after age 20). Strength training helps maintain muscle mass and increase your bone health, reducing the risk of osteoporosis. Strength training improves your ability to do everyday activities, like picking up your child or a bag of heavy groceries; these daily activities require strong muscles. More strength means you put less strain on your joints and reduce the risk of injuries.

BENEFITS OF METABOLIC TRAINING (BURN)

Metabolic training uses compound exercises with just a little rest in between exercises. This form of high-intensity training increases your metabolic rate during and after the workout. High-intensity workouts require more energy from anaerobic (that means without oxygen) pathways; the afterburn effect you get after working out like this is called EPOC (excess post-exercise oxygen consumption). Basically, you continue burning calories even when you are not working out! High-intensity interval training is efficient and effective, and I'm going to have you do a bit of it every day in your Wake-Up Workouts, but it's also challenging, so make sure to work at your own pace, especially if you're just getting started.

BENEFITS OF ATHLETIC TRAINING (BURN)

Athletic training requires us to move like our favorite sports players—we need agility, balance, speed, and coordination to perform these exercises. Agility is the ability to change the direction of the body quickly. Balance is our ability to maintain our equilibrium whether we're moving or standing still. Speed is movements such as sprinting and rapid jumps. Coordination is the ability to control the movement of your body in cooperation with the body's sensory functions, like catching a ball. I've designed particular Burn workouts to focus on specific skills in these categories.

BENEFITS OF CARDIO ENDURANCE TRAINING (SLOW BURN)

Steady-state cardio endurance training is a continuous aerobic activity. Examples include walking, jogging, biking, using an elliptical machine, or swimming. Unlike the metabolic and athletic training workouts that vary between high intensity and recovery intervals, steady-state training remains at a fixed intensity level. You move at a comfortable and moderate pace. Steady-state cardio work will increase your endurance and improve your mood. Anytime you're in a bad mood, get out and walk or do one of these activities if you possibly can, and you're likely to feel a lot better. This kind of aerobic exercise also reduces the risk of many health problems, including obesity, heart disease, high blood pressure, type 2 diabetes, and stroke.

BENEFITS OF FLEXIBILITY TRAINING (FLOW)

Flexibility is the ability of our joints and muscles to move through their full range of motion. Flexibility is primarily due to our genetics, but we all lose flexibility as we age and need to maintain it with regular training. Being flexible improves our posture, reduces the risk of injury, improves athletic performance, and can help reduce stress. The yoga flow that you will be doing is designed to not only increase your flexibility and range of motion, but also reduce stress and tension by helping you focus consciously on your breath.

The Program workouts have been designed to increase your fitness in all five of these areas and are balanced so that even though I'm asking you to work out every day, you shouldn't be straining or overusing any particular muscle area. The other cool thing about paying attention to these different ways of working out is you should get a more nuanced understanding of areas of your own fitness and how they vary. Most of us are stronger in one area or another, and most of you will find something to feel really good about, something that challenges you, and become more knowledgeable about which types of training support your specific goals.

BEFORE YOU BEGIN

Get a Checkup!

Before you begin any new exercise program, including The Program workouts, it is important that you check with your doctor and get a medical clearance to start exercising, especially if you haven't been active recently. Not all exercises are appropriate for everyone; you may need to modify some of the moves in The Program based on your personal health issues.

Monitor Your Intensity

You want to understand what you're going for in different types of workouts and how to have a sense of how hard you are working. One of the most common mistakes people make is not measuring their exercise intensity. You don't want to work too hard (which can lead to injury and burnout), or not work out hard enough (which can lead to frustration from lack of results). So keep track of your exercise intensity at every workout. The most common way to monitor exercise intensity is by target heart rate.

HEART RATE

To monitor your target heart rate, you can either wear a heart rate monitor or measure your pulse periodically as you exercise and stay within 50–85 percent of your maximum heart rate. This range is called your target heart rate. There are free target heart rate calculators online, or you can use the table below to calculate your target heart rate zone. According to the American Medical Association, your maximum heart rate is approximately 220 minus your age. Your target heart rate is generally between 50 and 75 percent of your maximum heart rate. If you choose to do any of your slow burn cardio walks or runs on a treadmill, most of these have heart monitor functions on them.

Moderate exercise intensity = 50–70 percent of your maximum heart rate
Vigorous exercise intensity = 70–85 percent of your maximum heart rate

If you're just starting out, aim for the lower end of your target zone (50 percent). Then, gradually increase your target zone.

MAXIMUM AND TRAINING HEART RATE, BY AGE

Age	Maximum Heart Rate per Minute	Training Zone: 60% Rate	Training Zone: 80% Rate
20	200	120	160
25	195	117	156
30	190	114	152
35	185	111	148
40	180	108	144
45	175	105	140
50	170	102	136
55	165	99	132
60	160	96	128
65	155	93	124

Source: American Medical Association

Some types of medications can lower your maximum heart rate and therefore lower your target heart rate zone. This is another good reason to check in with your doctor so you can ask if you need to use a lower target heart rate zone because of any medications you take or medical conditions you have.

FITNESS ASSESSMENTS

Your Training Schedule: Starting with Assessments

In addition to training in multiple ways, you want to train at an appropriate level. You don't want to hurt yourself. But once you get started, you do want to feel challenged. Your muscles and performance respond to appropriate training stress, which means you need to up the ante from one series of workouts to the next in order to see improvement; otherwise, your fitness will plateau. The beautiful thing is that your body is able to evolve and adapt to what you ask it to do. So be patient with your progress, but know that you need to push yourself. Listening to your body and finding that balance is key.

The first step on your 21-day transformation is to establish your fitness level in four key areas by taking some brief assessment tests. You might be having a not-so-pleasant flashback to your junior high school gym class right now, but don't worry, we're not grading these. My assessments are designed to give you an idea of what workouts are most appropriate to begin with and help you track your progress—you are in a judgment-free zone!

For the first 4 days of The Program, while Cleanse eating, you're going to perform a few brief exercises each morning to evaluate your fitness level in one key fitness area and follow up with a gentle slow cardio workout (walking, running, or some combination of the two) that is just meant to get you up and moving. The evaluations themselves are brief, so you can do the actual workout immediately following the fitness assessment, but you don't have to. It's fine to assess in the morning and work out at night if that fits your schedule. I like it when people can start their day with exercise, though, because you know you got it in and can carry that feeling through the day of having given yourself the gift of health.

Each fitness evaluation is a series of four exercises of the type I might have a new client do in my gym to figure out where they're at. Their main function for you is to help you figure out whether you should start training at the beginner, intermediate, or advanced level. But they are all solid exercises if you find you enjoy doing them and want to add them to your weekly routine going forward. And it's cool to track your progress using these exercises once in a while, too. You'll want to repeat the assessments at the end of your first cycle on The Program, and every month or so afterward, so you can change up your fitness goals as you need to and celebrate your progress.

Don't worry if it turns out you fall into different categories in different areas. You might be ready to do the advanced strength work out ("Full Throttle") but are more limited in your flexibility, so are doing the beginner series ("Getting Started") on that day. It's all good.

PEAK PERFORMANCE CONDITIONS

Finding the Right Challenge

It's important that people do something for movement every day. Some of the workouts you'll be doing on The Program are Tabata-influenced exercises, which are a form of high-intensity interval training (HIIT). These are brief and intense bursts of exercise that burn calories and boost your metabolism interspersed with periods of rest. You'll also need to try other new forms of exercise and strategies that get you excited to move.

You are reading this book, so I know you're motivated. It's time to take some action. You may have some very big goals, that's good, but can get overwhelming. Getting from here to there requires paying attention to one small decision at a time. It's easier for most people to think about making healthy choices while eating one meal at a time. Similarly, if you're feeling panicked about how far you have to go, just commit to one workout at a time. Worry about your next workout after you finish this one. Don't go too hard and burn out or get injured.

Some clients get excited about starting a new exercise program and think they need to do some cardio exercise and chase that "burn" feeling really hard. The enthusiasm is great, but if your muscles are not strong, you're going to wind up sore, worn out, and possibly too injured to do your next workout. That's no good. You want to follow a training plan that improves your core stability, strength, and agility, as well as your heart health, so you can get sweaty, sore, and tired in the right way, to see maximum results. That means you need to mix up your workouts, take the time to understand your own body's reaction to them, and, if necessary, slow down. Take things gradually.

Finding Partners

You'll read more about the importance of accountability in the "Connect" section of this book. While you do need to be accountable to other people, you do not absolutely need to work out with them. But there are tremendous benefits to exercising with a partner or a group, and I encourage you to seek out opportunities to do that during The Program. Consider starting The Program with a friend so you can support each other. Explore the possibility of trying a fitness class or group workout when you're challenged to find new ways to move. Working out with other people can provide motivation to show up, healthy competition to perform your best, friendship and encouragement from people who share your fitness goals, and, sometimes, inspiration from people who are a little ahead of you. Having an exercise partner keeps you accountable and can also make the time pass more enjoyably. Finally, taking a class or working with a professional trainer can be stimulating—it's an easy way to mix up your fitness routine and you can see new ways of doing things.

Don't be afraid to try out different gyms in your area if there are more than one. Gyms are like bars or other places that people gather: they have cultures. Most of them are very welcoming and thrilled to have people of all fitness levels, but one might feel more comfortable to you than another, so don't give up on gyms if you don't like the first one you visit. Explore your options. Sometimes going with a friend can make it less intimidating, too, so see if you can round up an interested partner.

I love the people at my gym, they make it feel like home to me. But gyms are not your only possible fitness community. Think about what you liked to do when you were a kid. Did you play basketball or soccer? Find an adult league. Did you like to bike? There might be a group of weekend riders in your area. Did you dance? Sign up for a class. You'll probably still like it. Was there something you always wanted to try? This is your moment to make it happen. As you try out new ways of moving on The Program, make some of it social if you can; you'll be much more likely to stick with it and you'll have more fun.

STAY IN MOTION

Walk

It might sound counterintuitive, but walking is a terrific choice if you're feeling tired and sore. Gentle movement of this kind will actually help you recover from most soreness more quickly than complete rest. It can also be energizing. If you're feeling restless and dying to keep moving, again, walking is great. Walking is not going to directly improve your performance at other activities, and it is not a tough enough exercise to build strength, but it is a low-to-no-impact way to burn calories, keep your blood flowing, and your muscles moving, all without generally impacting your ability to hit it hard during your next workout. Walking can also provide a restful mental reset. Little walks, long walks, it doesn't matter: it all adds up, and there's no downside to it. If in doubt, try walking it out.

Take the Stairs

You have heard this before, but, really, climbing stairs is great exercise and easy to fit into your day when you've got the choice between a few flights and an elevator. Fast, slow, skipping a stair in between—it's all good. Think of it as a little fitness bonus in your day every time you make this choice.

Take the Hill

If there is a choice between a flat road and a hilly one, take the time to walk, ride, or run up the hill once in a while. You don't have to be fast about it, and the hill doesn't have to be very steep. Even a gradual incline will work different muscles and challenge you in a way that you'll feel. The cool thing about this is that you usually feel a little stronger in your next regular (non-hilly) workout, especially if you make a hill a regular part of your routine.

Everything Counts

Look for ways to incorporate more activity into your day. Park farther away from your office entrance, take your dog for a longer walk, spend 20 minutes working in your yard or cleaning your apartment, throw a ball or go for a bike ride with your kids, meet a friend for coffee and a walk instead of sitting down at a table, do some stretching or weight work while you watch TV. You want to move more and you'll be surprised how naturally some of these things can fit into your life.

REST AND RECOVERY

People misunderstand the concept of recovery. Minor aches or soreness in your muscles after a workout are not necessarily bad. Take it easier when you feel them, but generally, gentle movement will help you recover better from this kind of soreness than doing nothing. If your legs ache after a run, take a walk or a yoga class the next day rather than skipping movement altogether. You'll generally feel better faster. To minimize soreness, make sure you take a few minutes to warm up before you work out. Don't skip over that part when you look at your Program plan.

During a hard workout, you need to rest and recover for a minute or more between tough efforts, exercises, or reps. After you work out, you want to refuel with protein and carbohydrates, rehydrate adequately, and preferably take time to stretch and/or strengthen your muscles, depending on what type of workout you did. You also want to alternate the types of training you do so that different muscles and systems in your body have a chance to rest, repair, and recover between workouts. This is when your body is really building and improving. The workouts on The Program are designed to help you find this balance.

Finally, your workouts will be most effective when you listen to your body. Your workouts should never be painful or make you sick. If you feel nauseous, dizzy, breathless, or faint while you're exercising, stop. Same goes if you experience pain in your chest, arms, neck, or jaw: stop. A good workout should make you feel the muscles you are working and build in time for recovery.

BONUS WORKOUT: STRETCH YOURSELF

Flexibility training is often overshadowed by cardiovascular and strength training, but if you want to train hard without injury, you need to incorporate flexibility training into your workouts. Sometimes people are confused about whether to stretch before or after working out, and this, plus impatience and time constraints, leads some to skip stretching altogether. That is a mistake. Please take my word for it, and don't wait for your body to let you know! The ideal time to work on flexibility training is right after you exercise, and it doesn't have to take a long time.

The key to proper stretching lies in the way you perform the stretch. When you're stretching certain parts of your body correctly, you should not feel pain. Staying relaxed is very important to stretching properly, and deep, easy, even breathing is the key to relaxation. If you notice yourself holding your breath while you are stretching, stop and start again. Your shoulders, hands, and feet should all be kept relaxed as you stretch. Make sure your body is not tight. Perform each stretch slowly and evenly. Hold the stretch for about 15 seconds and release slowly. Never bounce or jerk while stretching. This can cause injury if your muscle is pushed beyond its ability. All stretches should be smooth and slow. Flexibility exercises should be relaxing. Go slow and try to enjoy it!

Current guidelines from the American College of Sports Medicine recommend that stretching exercises for the major muscle groups be performed two or three times per week. Here are some basic stretches you should incorporate into your fitness program, whenever it is convenient for you.

Hamstrings

Setup: Stand shoulder-width apart, extend your right leg straight in front of you and bend your left knee.

Action: Keep your back long and lean forward from the hips over the straight leg. Make sure not to lock the right knee, keep it slightly bent. Your hands should rest on your bent knee. Stop when you feel a pull in the hamstring. Hold for 30 seconds. Repeat with the other leg.

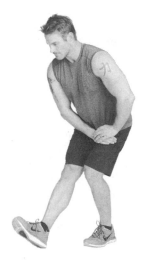

Quadriceps

Setup: Stand on your left foot and grasp your right shoelaces.

Action: Tuck your pelvis in and gently pull your heel to your glutes. Hold for 30 seconds.

Repeat with the other leg. *Use a sturdy chair or table if you need help balancing.

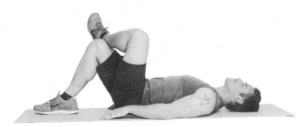

Glutes and Hips

Setup: Lie on your back, with legs extended. Bend your left knee and place your right ankle on your left thigh.

Action: With both hands gently pull the bent knee toward your chest. Hold for 30 seconds.

Repeat with the other leg.

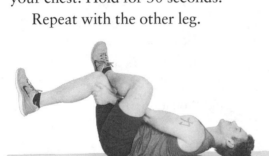

Chest Openers

Setup: Stand with your arms crossed at chest level.

Action: Open your arms out and back, feeling your chest and shoulders. Hold for two breaths.

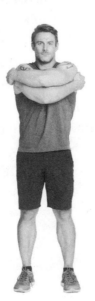

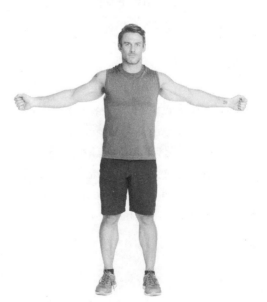

Sleep

It almost goes without saying that you will perform your best when you are well rested. The problems associated with being chronically overtired are both mental and physical, and will impact your appetite, your hormones, your stress level, and well as the way your body processes food. Most adults need 7 to 8 hours of sleep each day. If you have trouble getting enough sleep, make it a priority to improve.

It helps to wake up and go to bed at a consistent time every day, which depends on your schedule and, optimally, your own body rhythms. Try making your bedroom relatively cool, as lightproof as possible, and don't have any screens (TV, computers, phones, etc.) in there if you can help it. If that's unavoidable, try limiting your use of them before bedtime, preferably shutting everything down at least an hour or two before you go to sleep. Once you start moving more, hopefully it'll help you sleep as well. If you start getting adequate sleep, you'll really notice a difference when you work out.

PRACTICAL DETAILS

Plan Ahead

We make time for the things that are important. You are important and so is giving yourself the gift of health. Prioritize it. After the 4-day Cleanse period, you're going to need to find about 45 minutes in your day to devote to exercise going forward. These minutes do not need to be consecutive, but they do need to be planned for. I know it's appealing to see a fitness program that promises big changes from only 10 minutes of exercise a day. This is not that. While little things add up and some movement is better than no movement, if you want to see significant results, you're going to need to make a significant effort. So get out your calendar and schedule your workout time. For some of you, that might mean setting the alarm clock a half hour earlier. For others, it might mean spending your lunch hour differently a few times a week; still others may need to figure out a child care swap with a friend. Whatever it is you need to do to facilitate the time for exercise, it's worth it. You may even find you start to look forward to it.

There are certain exercises you can do while you're multitasking, like watching TV. Sometimes it helps to break up your workouts into smaller chunks during the day. You may need to switch up your exercise time on different days of the week—most people do. Try a bunch of different strategies, and whatever works for you, make it nonnegotiable.

What to Wear

If you are motivated by having new or special workout clothes, knock yourself out. But you really don't need to wear anything special to do these workouts. Loose, comfortable, stretchy shirts, shorts, or pants that don't get in your way are all fine. Some people prefer the feeling of a technical, sweat-wicking fabric to a cotton T-shirt, but the choice is yours. Do get a decent pair of sneakers. Some of the exercises could be done barefoot, but I generally recommend that my clients wear supportive sneakers for working out. Take a few minutes to have everything you need right in front of you when you get up in the morning, so you can move right into your Wake-Up Workouts once they start.

Fitness Terms

SETS AND REPS

You will see the terms *sets* and *reps* on the instructions for your strength training workouts. A set is a group of successive repetitions performed with no rest between the exercises. You might be asked to do four different exercises in a set. *Rep* is short for *repetition*, the number of times you repeat an exercise in each set. You might be asked to repeat a particular exercise five times (5 reps) before moving on to the next one in the set.

Example: If I ask you to do three sets of 12 reps of push-ups, you would do 12 push-ups (first set), rest, then complete 12 more push-ups (second set), rest again, and finish with 12 more push-ups (third set).

INTERVAL TRAINING

Your athletic training workouts and metabolic training workouts give you a specific amount of time to perform the exercises and a specific amount of time to rest. This is high-intensity interval training, and you are meant to really push yourself to get the correct number of reps done in time, then rest just enough to recover and do it again. This gets your heart rate up, boosts your metabolism, and makes for a very effective, efficient use of your workout time. One form of interval training is Tabata, which consists of 20 seconds of work and 10 seconds of rest, repeated for 4 minutes. The Program workouts in these areas are designed to introduce you to this style of working out. They are challenging, but also brief. You can do it!

COOL-DOWN

The cool-down is simply doing something easy, like walking or stepping in place, for a bit instead of abruptly stopping after exercise. Stopping exercising suddenly can cause dizziness. You want to spend a few minutes in gentle motion to let your heart rate return to normal. The blood vessels in your legs expand during strenuous exercise, which brings more blood to your legs and feet. If you stop exercising too suddenly, your heart rate slows quickly and that blood can pool in your lower body and cause you to feel dizzy or even faint. So don't just sit down when you complete your sets, take a few moments at the end of your workout to cool down.

EQUIPMENT FOR THE WORKOUTS

Ideally you will have a mat, some dumbbells, a bench or a sturdy chair, resistance bands, and a stability ball. This equipment will give you a mini home gym and allow you to progress to more challenging exercises. But you can start The Program with only a mat and a pair of dumbbells.

RESISTANCE BANDS

Resistance bands are great because they are cheap, compact, portable, and versatile.

They are so compact and lightweight that you can easily take them along when you travel or if you want to do a quick a workout at the office.

Resistance bands generally come in three or four different levels of resistance and cost about $15 per band. Look for bands that come with a door anchor attachment. Choose the appropriate level of resistance for you; the exercises that use the bands can be used with any of them.

STABILITY BALL (SWISS, BALANCE, STRETCH, AND PHYSIO BALL)

It doesn't really matter what you call it, just as long as you use it! Stability balls can provide a great upper-body workout, a lower-body workout, and a challenging abdominal workout, and they can assist your stretching. How many things improve your balance and posture merely by sitting on them? Because the stability ball is an unstable surface, you have to use all of your stability muscles in your core just to balance. You can also use the stability ball as a weight bench.

Stability balls are usually sold in three sizes. Purchase the stability ball based on your height:

4'11"–5'4" = 55 centimeter ball
5'4"–5'11" = 56 centimeter ball
5'11" and up = 75 centimeter ball

DUMBBELLS

Dumbbells are usually sold in pairs, or you can purchase an all-in-one variety, such as Powerblock, which has options from 5 to 50 pounds. The all-in-one options are more expensive and may not be necessary, depending on your fitness level. To start out you just need one light pair of dumbbells and a heavy pair. For most women, pairs of 5- and 10-pound weights will get you started, and for men, pairs of 15- and 25-pound dumbbells might be a good starting point. But try them before you buy them.

When you use weights for strength-building exercises, you want them to be heavy enough to challenge your muscles to burn. That means, in general, that you should be lifting enough weight so that you are struggling to finish the last repetition of each set. For example, if you are doing biceps curls with 10-pound dumbbells and at the end of the first set of 12 reps you feel like you could do five more reps, you want to try increasing the weight to 12 or 15 pounds.

WEIGHT BENCHES OR STEPS

You will be lying on the bench or step for some of the upper body exercises and using it for leg exercises (step-ups and jumps), so the higher your bench or step is, the more challenging the exercise will be. The bench or step should ideally be high enough that when you step on it your knee is at a 90-degree angle.

You can find all of these items online and at local sporting goods stores. You may want to check out a used sporting goods store in your area; they usually have great deals on all the equipment you'll need.

Focus on Form

The most important thing to focus on during all of your workouts is your form. Some people focus on the quantity of their reps and sets as opposed to the quality of each exercise. Pay attention to your form, especially at the beginning if these exercises are new to you, and maybe do a practice few before starting the sets to make sure you understand the goal of the exercise. If you find during the set that you need to take a break or do fewer reps in order to maintain good form, do it, because that is always better than continuing the exercise with poor form.

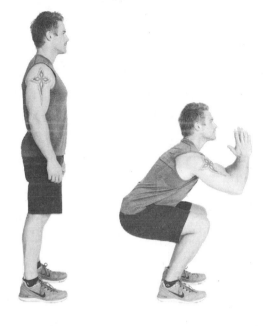

THE SQUAT

Keep your chest open.

Keep your core tight.

Keep your back straight, with a neutral spine.

Lower to 90 degrees. If you don't complete the full range of motion, you are not fully engaging your glutes and hamstrings.

Your weight should be on the heels and balls of your feet.

THE DEAD LIFT

Bend at your hip joint, not at your waist.

Look forward.

Don't round your back.

Keep dumbbells close to your legs.

Squeeze your glutes to pull yourself up.

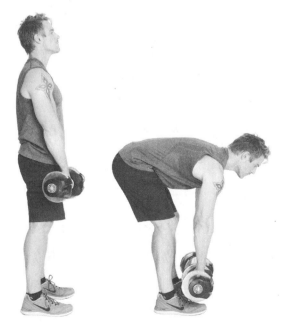

THE PUSH-UP

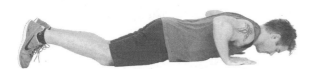

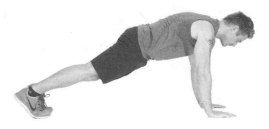

Keep your head in a neutral position.

Place your hands straight on the floor, fingers pointed forward.

Keep your elbows in (don't flare).

Tighten your abs and squeeze your glutes.

DUMBELL ROWS

Keep your chest open.

Keep a straight line from the top of your head to your tailbone.

Tighten your abs.

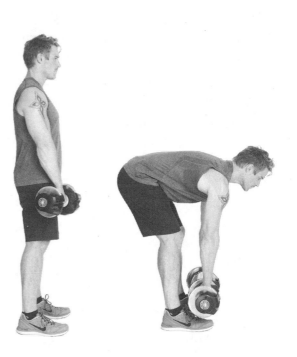

Set goals to get results

You don't want to spin your wheels at the gym. It's fine to want to be thinner, and your weight management can be a motivating goal to get you to work out. But I think it helps to figure out if you want to be fitter, stronger, healthier, more flexible, and/or more agile and can measure your progress on those terms in realistic ways. Having smaller goals—like *I want to be able to lift this much weight or do this many reps of that exercise or walk this many miles*—will help you focus your attention and make the most of your physical training.

Take a breath!

We all know how to breathe, right? You're doing it right now, without even thinking about it, but when you exercise you *need* to think about how to breathe. We all have different instincts about breathing when we work out, and most of them do not support an optimal performance. I've worked with people who hold their breath when they are doing high-intensity workouts and others who are breathing quickly before they even warm up. Here are the breathing strategies to keep in mind during all of your workouts:

Strength training: You want to inhale on the less strenuous phase and exhale on the hardest part of the exercise. As an example, when you do a push-up, you want to exhale as you push yourself up and inhale as you lower down.

Athletic/metabolic high-intensity training: During high-intensity training, your breath should come from the diaphragm, not the chest. That means that when the level of intensity ramps up, you should inhale through your nose and exhale through your mouth. These are demanding cardio intervals, and they can leave you breathless, so be sure to take calm, deep breaths during the recovery intervals.

Slow burn cardio: During steady state cardio workouts, your goal should be to maintain continuous breathing in a comfortable manner. In other words, you should be able to have a conversation with someone while you're moving.

Flexibility: Try to take your inhales and exhales in equal lengths; slow deep breathing can increase your ability to go deeper into your stretches. Your nerves control the stretch reflex, and when your body senses that a muscle is being stretched beyond its normal range of motion, your nerves will signal the muscles to contract in order to protect the muscles from damage. You can delay that stretch reflex by breathing deeply and exhaling into the stretch, then you're better able to hold the stretch longer. Try to maintain each stretch for 30–45 seconds. Remember not to stretch a cold muscle; this kind of stretching should be performed after your workouts, not before.

Think

At the beginning of this book, I told you it's important to figure out your Why. It will strengthen your commitment and increase your energy to succeed, and it makes it easier to keep on track if things feel like a grind. Identifying and understanding your Why requires self-awareness. There are practical things you can do to cultivate awareness in your life.

I believe that we all wake up every morning with full power. We're full of potential to be our best and make it a great day. Then we get busy. We tend to spend our days zooming through our to-do lists, running from one task or obligation to another, taking care of others, and trying to fit everything in. This is the reality of most of our everyday lives. The problem is that when we don't make time to stop and pay attention to why and how we're doing all the things we do, we lose our sense of purpose and meaning and, often, our power. When that happens, a lot of us engage in behaviors that start to make us feel stuck, anxious, and stressed out, and we don't even realize we're doing it. Or maybe we see ourselves doing them and know it's unproductive but don't know how to stop. The Program requires you to take time to stop and pay attention to yourself, accept where you are, and figure out how to get where you need to be.

I know that there are a lot of people and things in your life worthy of your attention. But you're one of them. When you put everyone else's needs in front of your own—those of your kids, your spouse, your boss, your pet, your parents—no one gets the best of you. I've found that a lot of my clients struggle with making time for this kind of self-care. It is not selfish to meet your own needs, and it will benefit everyone around you. Ultimately it means taking responsibility for yourself.

During The Program, you are going to create a routine of healthy mind rituals and see how you feel after practicing them for one cycle. Everyone is different, so you'll want to give each practice a chance and evaluate what worked best for you, what didn't, and why. But most people find some of these practices keep them focused on their eating and training goals. By the way, you don't have to be in any kind of distress to benefit from these practices. Think of them as tools in your toolbox to help you be a little happier. Or like secret weapons for getting fit and living well.

There are four ways you'll be harnessing your mind power during The Program: Set intentions. Breathe. Pay attention. Be grateful. These don't have to take a lot of time, so I'm going to ask you to employ some form of all four of them every day.

SET INTENTIONS

If you have any experience practicing yoga, you may have come across the idea of setting an intention. I want you to set an intention for the day each morning. This is a loose idea, at least the way I want you to use it. It can be a dedication, an attitude, a wish, a mission statement, an inspirational quote, a focal point—anything that sets the tone for how you want your day to unfold. Think of your intention as a seed, a kind of potential, that has the power to grow into something big as you cultivate and nurture it.

Intentions are not the same as goals, but they can help guide you toward your goals. Name your goals. They can and should be both large and small. Why are you doing The Program? What do you want to change about your body or your life? What do you want to accomplish in the next week? In the next month? The next year?

Some people find this process really uncomfortable. Do it anyway. Don't be superstitious, afraid of failing, or scared to say your goals out loud or write them down. Admit them to yourself. Don't expect to achieve them overnight. My clients who are able to maintain weight loss and a healthy lifestyle understand that setting goals means you risk disappointing yourself and that you improve the possibility of learning from yourself and figuring out how to do better tomorrow. Once you have set some goals for yourself and are ready to start The Program, you'll want to take a minute or two each morning on The Program to set an intention for the day that helps you stay on track towards those goals.

Remember, this is not a to-do list; it's a way to bring focus and meaning to the start of your day. You don't have to write it down, but I think it helps. You can jot it as a note on your phone, send an email to yourself, write it out in a notebook dedicated to this practice—whatever works for you. Intentions are extremely personal. Examples of intentions people have shared with me include:

"I am going to get up and move today."

"Today I'm going to say I can."

"I am going to be brave today."

"I am strong."

"I am lovable."

"I am loved."

"I am good."

"I am beautiful."

"I will earn my body today."

"I'm going to go the extra mile today."

"I am worth it."

I want you to try this even if it feels weird or awkward. It is a small thing that I have seen be a powerfully effective tool to keep people on track when they are establishing new habits. There are other ways to do it. You might find your daily intention in a photograph of a place or person you love, or one that reminds you of somewhere (or a state of mind) that you want to be. Visualizing is a common training tool for athletes. They visualize themselves performing correctly over and over, and when they train, they visualize themselves getting stronger and reaching a specific goal. You can do this, too. And it doesn't have to just be in your imagination. Having a picture of yourself that you like or of someone or something that inspires you or reminds you of where you want to be can be a good motivator. I have a client who uses images to set her intentions, and she will take a screen shot of something inspiring to look at and set it on the lock screen on her phone each day. Figure out what motivates you or what you're excited about for the day and take a minute to set your focus.

Being conscious of your intentions is a crucial component of living well. It is so important to be positive, to focus on the healthy behaviors you are engaging in and the reasons why you're changing. Every day is a new day and another opportunity to do it better. Setting intentions helps to remind yourself of that, and is even more important after those days when you are inevitably going to make choices you regret. If you screwed up last night, move forward. Notice how you felt. You need to remember that feeling and use it to stay powerful in the new day when setting your new intention.

Going the extra mile: If you find you have time in the morning and enjoy the process of writing, you can expand on the morning intention and write in more detail about how you're feeling and what you're excited about. Don't feel pressured to do that; setting the intention is enough. But some people want to go deeper. Vision boards also work for certain people. This is a bulletin or poster board where you display or arrange images that represent where you want to be in any or all areas of your life. Think of it as a kind of visual map of photographs, drawings, quotations, or anything else that inspires you and connects you with your dreams. If you are the crafty type, go for it and make one, then look at it purposefully in the morning or just have it around where your subconscious mind can take it in. Visualizing success can reinforce your intentions and your willpower.

BREATHE

So many things compete for our time, fragmenting our concentration. It's easy to become distracted and overwhelmed. Focusing on your breath is a quick and effective technique both for calming down and for helping to remind you of your own priorities, whatever they are. As you go through your day and take a bit of a beating here and there, eroding your goodwill and motivation, remember that you can shut your eyes, breathe deeply, and not let everything simply happen to you.

Obviously you're breathing all the time without thinking about it. But as you start to reconnect with yourself as a physical being you'll be paying more conscious attention to your breath. There are specific techniques you can use for breathing while you're working out, as I covered in the "Sweat" section of this book, but I'm talking about something different here.

Take a moment to stop during the day, especially if you find yourself feeling stressed, and focus on your breathing. You might be surprised at how often you discover yourself holding your breath. It's a subconscious way of attempting to control emotion and anxiety. That takes energy. If you notice that you're doing it, just take a long inhale and exhale, and repeat. You'll figure out what feels comfortable for you, but if you're having trouble, I once heard someone describe this to a child as "Picture yourself holding a piece of hot pizza. Smell the pizza, then blow on the pizza." The point is just to take a moment and breathe very consciously.

As your mind wanders all over the place, as it inevitably will, try simply concentrating on your breath. You don't have to do this for a long time: you can take 10 or 20 deep breaths and think of yourself as recharging in a moment. That's it. I think of this as both a way of keeping your power and also, sometimes, giving yourself important information about your state of mind.

Practices that have us tune into our breath and calm down can help reduce stress and blood pressure, and strengthen the immune system. Most of us live in our heads more than our bodies, and we don't tune into ourselves physically: we either pay no attention when things are going well or want to block out painful physical sensations or emotions. But our bodies have so much to tell us about how we're doing, both physically and emotionally. When you deliberately pay attention to yours, starting with your breath, you'll be better able to see how particular things are affecting you.

Breathing consciously also shifts things. It can help you detach from your emotions even as you tune in and notice them. Finally, breathing can also give us a good clue to our state of mind when we pay attention to it. You might notice that it changes and calms while—and just because—you're paying attention to it. Think of paying attention to your breath as a quick way of shifting gears when you start to feel overwhelmed. You can do this in the car, at your desk, in the bathroom—literally any time you need to take a minute. It doesn't have to be on any kind of schedule, and no one needs to know you're doing it.

Going the extra mile: There are a lot of specific breathing techniques you can explore to use in different situations. One that many people find effective when they need to harness energy or focus is called alternate nostril breathing, which might sound strange but is worth a try. When you're sitting comfortably, use your right thumb to press your right nostril closed and inhale deeply in through your left nostril. At the peak of that inhale, use your right index finger to close off the left nostril, release your thumb and exhale through your right nostril. Repeat this pattern a few times, continuing to inhale through the right side of your nose and exhaling through the left side, and see if you don't feel more clear. If you find that doing different breathing techniques helps you, know that this is only one of many brief, directed breathing exercises you can try.

PAY ATTENTION

In addition to getting into the habit of paying attention to your breath in order to stay calm and tune into your body, you also want to cultivate a habit of paying attention to your thoughts. Starting The Program means you've set goals for yourself, and you need to harness your mind power to achieve those goals. The messages we give ourselves every day are a kind of energy and force, and yet we tend not to be mindful about them.

Being mindful means paying attention to things you wouldn't normally notice, and I want you to get into the habit of setting aside some time each day to deliberately pay some calm attention to your own experience as it unfolds, without judgment. Tuning into where you're at in the moment requires taking a few minutes to be purposefully conscious of your mind and body. There are several ways to do this, and I want you to try them out as they fit your schedule. But try them all over the course of The Program.

If you have 5 minutes today, stop whatever you are doing. Close the door, shut your phone off (or set a 5 minute timer on it), stop moving, and withdraw. Close your eyes. Allow the cascade of thoughts in your mind to settle. This takes time and can feel uncomfortable. You are not sleeping or resting. Don't try to control what your mind is thinking. Stay still and notice your feelings and experiences. Don't worry about why you're having particular thoughts or what to do about them, just notice them. Don't judge them. There is no right or wrong.

Do you notice any physical sensations in your body? Where are they? What are they like? Do you feel a particular emotion? How do you know you're experiencing it? Do you feel it physically? What thoughts are you having? Again, simply notice whatever comes to mind and let it flow by. There is no need to try to analyze, understand, or change any of your observations; just notice them. When 5 minutes has passed, you can stop and move forward with your day.

If you have 15 minutes today, shut your phone off (or set a timer) and find a quiet space. You can sit on a chair or on the floor, lie down or stand up, in whatever position feels comfortable—but maybe not lying on your bed or the couch, because you don't want to be so relaxed that you fall asleep. Get comfortable, close your eyes, and take a few deep breaths. Don't try to filter any thoughts, noise, or other sensations; simply notice them and try to focus on your breath. Some people find it helps to focus on their breath moving through a specific body part as they do this, either their nose, chest, belly, or mouth. That's it. When your mind wanders, simply notice the thought and redirect your attention to the in and out of your breathing.

Other people find visualizing an image helps them stay focused on the breath. A common one is to imagine a small light in the center of your breastbone. As you inhale, imagine that light expanding. As you exhale, imagine the light receding back to its original small size. Repeat. That's it. It's another technique to help you stay focused on your breathing, so when your mind wanders, you can bring it back to the breath and the image of the light.

If you are thinking, "Jessie, you've got to be kidding; I have no extra time today," you are not off the hook! Another way of practicing mindfulness is by observing yourself experiencing a small task. So try really paying attention to something you might normally do unconsciously. The classic example is washing the dishes; another one is folding the laundry. Instead of multitasking and watching a TV show or talking on your phone while you fold the laundry, try giving this chore your full attention and notice all your senses and bodily sensations as you experience it. What do the clean clothes smell like? How do the different fabrics and textures feel in your hands? How are you feeling as you fold? Are you hunching your shoulders? In other words, give this chore your complete attention. As with the other mindful practices, try not to judge or change any of these thoughts, just be with them. If it's not laundry day, you can try doing this when you brush your teeth—I know you're fitting that in, or at least I hope you are.

You might be wondering how this all this fits into your physical fitness goals. In addition to its other benefits, being mindful in this meditative way helps you practice discipline and willpower. When I am doing these types of exercises, I often find myself thinking about things I need to do. I remember obligations that feel urgent, like an email I forgot to respond to or a call I promised to make. Those tasks are real and I want or have to do them, or at least write them down so I don't forget about them. But in that moment that I am thinking about them, instead I wait, because I have made a decision to make space for mindfulness, so whatever I'm remembering needs to keep for 15 minutes. Every time I do this it gets easier. Now, there may be times when you feel an urgent need to snack or eat, or an impulse to mindlessly eat food at work or a party when you aren't actually hungry. Because you are pausing for a few minutes in one area, you may find it easier to pause in this other area, to stop and say to yourself, *Okay, I notice that impulse, let me get back to it in 5 or 10 minutes.* You're breaking the habit of needing to act on your impulses immediately and being mindful about the action you are about to take.

Going the extra mile: I have you exploring some meditative exercises, but there are a ton of ways to actually practice meditation if you find that you like it. Some of them can be physical, like yoga or tai chi, qi gong, labyrinth walking, and certain kinds of dance. There are other ways of meditating that are totally stationary. There are silent styles of meditation, and others that involve chanting, candles, music, or someone else guiding you with words. These all work, and some might be more comfortable for you than others. If you're interested, consider exploring other types of meditation practices, either through what's available in your community or through books and tapes in your library. There are also some cool meditation resources available online, including on my website JessiePavelka.com; feel free to use it to explore what is most effective for you.

BE GRATEFUL

At night, we tend to think we had a "good day" or a "bad day," and that's if we haven't already moved right on to our list of things we need to get done tomorrow. The truth is that you had a bunch of different moments and experiences today. Take a minute at the end of the day and pick three things that made you happy or that you can feel grateful for. Write them down in a notebook or a file on your computer or phone dedicated to this purpose. You are going to do this throughout The Program. Some days it will be easy, and other days you might have to dig a little, but it shouldn't take you more than a minute or two, and I guarantee that if you think about it, you will find at least three moments to be grateful for each night.

What you write each day should be specific but does not need to be detailed. They can be major milestones or fleeting moments. Some examples of things people have shared with me from their gratitude lists include:

"Hydrangeas blooming in yard today."
"Ate a perfect peach."
"Pushing my kids on the swings at the park."
"Walked after dinner."
"Loving new book that I started today."
"Email from my son."
"Saw amazing sunrise when walking the dog."
"Did record number of push-ups in 60 seconds."
"My hair looked really good."
"Made it to the gym after all."

You get the idea. You're stopping to be aware of what went right today, and it's okay if those things were small. This will help you to be conscious of the things you have to be grateful for, the things that bring you satisfaction, and the things that engage and inspire you.

You want to keep this in a list format because it's helpful to notice patterns when you have been doing this for a little while. If you see that going for a walk after dinner is often making you happy, or that getting up early enough to see the sun rise made your list three times over a couple weeks, maybe you should try to do those things more often. Many people are surprised at how often movement-based activity turns out to be a high point of their day, and recording it encourages them to do it more often. Whatever it is that's making you happy, keep doing it.

The other great thing about recording the things that make you happy is that you can flip back when you're feeling low or discouraged and see how much you have to be grateful for in the big picture. Many people find it satisfying to look at their lists as they get longer; it helps them get perspective and celebrate the good stuff. Also, you might find that the habit of doing this makes you more tuned into those moments when they are actually happening. Notice what they feel like. You don't have to try to create them. They are already happening to you.

Going the extra mile: Another form of list making that some of my clients find helpful is to keep a training journal, a record specifically devoted to their physical training. They take a couple minutes to record the amount of time or distance they walked each day, or how many push-ups they did, or miles they biked, and they note any unusual details about the workout. People who like doing this find it satisfying to review their progress and notice patterns over time to help them train more effectively. Other people find it stressful to keep track of their numbers this way. It's definitely not for everyone. Try it if you think you might find it motivating. If you decide to keep a training journal, I recommend keeping it as a separate file or notebook from your gratitude list.

HARNESSING YOUR MIND POWER

All four of the Think practices I've asked you to try for the duration of The Program can be done in 5 minutes or less. While you can benefit from spending more time on some of them, you don't have to, and the potential payoff for less than 20 minutes a day is tremendous. You may experience some relaxation or have an important insight during some of these exercises, and if you do, that's great, but don't feel like these are goal oriented. There's no failing, and there's rarely an ultimate victory. There will probably not be a moment where you say to yourself, *I'm amazing, I'm conscious, grateful, and totally in tune with the universe.* (If you have one, let me know how you did it!) The goal of these exercises is to help you become more in tune with yourself and to use that knowledge to help your physical training and self-discipline in several ways.

As you pay attention to your thoughts, you can eventually redirect the unproductive ones and change your experience. When you are actively slowing down to do these exercises, you don't want to judge your thoughts or respond to them. Just notice them and let them pass. But pay attention. Are some of your thoughts repetitive? Defeating? Negative? Distracting? A lot of us find it so uncomfortable to have those kinds of thoughts that we do unhelpful things—like unnecessary eating or drinking—to avoid them. You'll be developing the discipline to simply sit with those kinds of feelings during some of these exercises.

Many people who have struggled with their weight or fitness have self-defeating thoughts about their ability to become healthier. If you find that you are nervous about whether you can be successful, these Think exercises can help you get comfortable with accepting the idea of failure. If this is you, here's the thing: if you're scared, accept it. You might fail. It's a possibility. A lot of trainers will tell you that when you think you can't do something, you need to change your attitude; that if you accept failure as a possibility, you will fail. This is a "refuse to lose" mentality. I'm going to go ahead and say that transformation is scary, and yes, you might fail. Acknowledge it, accept it, and decide you want to go for it anyway, and see what happens. The practice of actively noticing your feelings teaches you not to resist anxious or uncomfortable feelings. Just accept that you have them and let them exist while you take action. This is more of a "feel the fear and do it anyway" philosophy.

Everything you need to be successful exists inside you right now. When you use discipline to build strength and clarity in your mind, you are moving toward feeling better in your body. When you use your mind power to stick to actions that bring you closer to your intentions, you are moving toward feeling in control and being happier. These possibilities are worth 20 minutes of your day.

Connect

Your success in reaching your goals depends on your taking responsibility for your own health and fitness. But you don't have to do it alone, and you shouldn't. The quality of your relationships impacts your happiness and well-being, your motivation and performance, and your accountability and health. Taking some time to pay attention to four key relationships and cultivate some healthy ones is part of The Program.

The Connect practices are different from your Think exercises. I don't expect you to be taking intentional time for all four of your major relationship areas every day, although you are going to want an accountability partner that you check in with pretty regularly. But after reviewing this section, I'd like you to commit to taking one action each day to enhance one of these relationships and to work on connecting in all four of these areas of your life for the duration of The Program.

SELF

Let's start with an important relationship that most people overlook: the one you have with yourself. When you do some of the exercises in the Think section of The Program, you'll be starting to tune in a bit more to your experience, both physical and emotional. The practice I want you to try here is somewhat different, because rather than simply acknowledging your feelings and getting comfortable with the tough ones, you're going to try taking some action to challenge them, in order to connect—or reconnect—with your best self.

Our thoughts dictate our moods. Everything starts with a thought. When you pay attention to the thought patterns that you are allowing to run through your head, it will give you some insight into what makes you feel a certain way, and if you can redirect the negative thoughts, it may help you to become a stronger, more self-loving person.

Change the thought pattern, change the feeling. It really is that simple. If you don't like what you are watching on the TV or listening to on the radio, what do you do?

You pick up the remote and change the channel, right? You can learn to do the same with your thought patterns.

Look at Yourself. And Listen.

Set some time aside when you can be alone and look at yourself in a mirror. A full-length mirror is ideal, but if you want or need to use a smaller one it's okay. Really look into your own eyes, look at your face and body, and think about where you have been and what you want for yourself. Stay still and look for longer than you want to, maybe 5 full minutes. Most people find this to be a very weird and uncomfortable experience, but it's important. I find that it generally triggers challenging and helpful insights.

You might not like what you see. That's okay. Tell yourself this is Day 1, and keep looking. I worked with a client, Sara, who did the exercise with me in the room. I asked her what she saw in the mirror and she said, "I hate myself."

I told Sara that nothing was going to change until she started loving herself, and I asked her to think of some good things about herself. You should do this, too, if you're not already doing it naturally. If you find it difficult to identify things about your physical being that you can feel good about, focus on your experience as a person. Think about things you may have overcome or endured, experiences that made you feel powerful and strong. I have worked with people who were in very low places, emotionally and physically. I had a client struggle for something good to say about himself until he finally came up with "I guess I'm still here."

If that's where you are, hold on to that thing, whatever it is that gives you a bit of power. It can be something about your body, such as liking the way your smile or your eyes look; it can be a memory of a physical triumph, like running a race or giving birth to your child; it can be the knowledge that you've endured something painful and are still here, like the loss of a job or the death of a family member. The point is that you are reestablishing a relationship with yourself that needs to be honest and kind, in the same way that you would hope your best relationships with other people would be. You may need to change the conversation with yourself. To that end, you want to notice the way you observe yourself and try reframing some of your negative observations:

"My legs are too big" can become "My legs are strong."
"My arms are sore" can become "My arms are changing and getting stronger."
"I've got a long way to go" can become "I'm worth the struggle."

You get the idea. If it helps, think about what you would say if you heard a friend you cared about say something self-defeating. You would, hopefully, be honest in your response but also encouraging and optimistic. Show yourself the same care and repeat this exercise with the mirror once a week throughout The Program.

Know Your Negatives

The catalyst for a lot of my clients are feelings of self-loathing. They just can't stand to look—or live—a particular way any longer. Here's the problem: maybe that gets someone started, but you won't sustain your changes without changing your outlook.

We all have places in ourselves that we tend to feel self-conscious or unhappy about. You don't want those negative thoughts to transform into destructive behavior patterns that make you feel out of control. Sometimes I ask people to give themselves 10 minutes on the clock—no longer—and just write down all the negative thoughts that they are struggling with, even if they seem crazy. When the time is up, take a deep breath, review your list, and respond to it in a rational, positive way. Try to reframe your fear as excitement and see the opportunities in your obstacles. Try to focus on the things your body can do as opposed to the parts of it you want to change.

Remember—or Rediscover—What Makes You Happy

Many clients who start The Program find that moving their bodies again makes them happy. Maybe the actual time in the gym is painful—although more people than you'd expect really start to look forward to some parts of their workout—but almost everyone finds that post-exercise feeling to be a source of pleasure. For some, this is a new discovery; for others, it's a reminder of a feeling they had as a student athlete or just a kid running around being physical.

What other experiences, either in your past or in your dreams, do you want to explore? I think that in the same way we all have bodies that are designed to move, we all have an instinct to be creative in some way that can bring us pleasure and happiness if we can tap into it. My dad plays in a band, so I grew up surrounded by music, but I didn't pick up an instrument until I was 25, when I taught myself to play the guitar. Now, I'm not ready to go out in public with it, but I find playing and writing music to be a really satisfying outlet. It makes me feel good when I'm sad and allows me to use my brain and body in ways that are completely different from how I spend most of my working days.

Do you have a creative outlet like this? Don't think about it too much. Just consider something that excites you and tap into the process. You can reconnect with a skill or interest that you have, or try something that's completely new. I have clients who paint, draw, make music, knit, sew, cook, and carve. And you don't have to have any kind of agenda or improvement plan in this area. This is about the process, not the end result. If you try, for example, drawing with a pencil and paper for an hour one night this week instead of watching TV, whatever you wind up with is entirely beside the point. The goal is just to immerse yourself, however briefly, in the meditative process of making something.

Don't just dream about your creativity, take action. Write down three things you liked to do when you were a kid. Let's say you liked to read, ride your bike, and color. Do them this week. Alternatively, think about three things you've always wanted to learn how to do. Maybe that's painting, playing an instrument, or learning another language. Pick one and make a plan to try it out.

Doing Small Things Differently

Another way of reconnecting with yourself is by shaking up your routine in small ways. The Program requires you to make changes in the way you eat and schedule movement into your day. Be open to experiencing other aspects of your life differently as well. Take a different route to work. Work out at different times of the day and night. Make one meal of foods that are entirely new to you. Go someplace new in your town. You get the idea. These changes don't have to be a big deal. But doing things a little differently will usually make you more conscious of the things around you. Think about the difference in the quality of your attention when you drive a route that you are very familiar with compared with one that you've never done before. You're more alert and watchful, usually, if you have to take a new path. You want to cultivate this quality of wakefulness in your life in general.

A HIGHER POWER

We all have moments when life seems overwhelming. For some of my clients, overeating has been a way of getting through the day. When you are struggling to believe in your own ability to take care of yourself, you need supportive relationships. For many people, having a belief in something outside of yourself, something higher than yourself, is a useful way of confronting the tough moments, keeping things in perspective, and making better choices.

It can be helpful if there is something or someone that you feel you can hand your stress and anxiety over to. I grew up in a religious home and have seen the great things that faith can do for people. Some of my clients have found religious faith to be a significant source of strength, inspiration, and support as they struggle to make changes in their lives. Everyone's relationship to their faith is different, but one thing I've noticed is that worship services tend to have moments of complete stillness that are rare in most of our lives. We don't generally make a lot of room for silence, reflection, and time for just "being" instead of "doing."

You don't have to be a practicing member of a particular religion to have those moments. When I was a boy, I played outside all day long, and I continue to feel very connected to nature. As an adult, I've realized that it's possible to feel connected to something greater than me, and to feel God when I am outdoors. I think being outside, in nature, especially early in the morning in a beautiful place, can help remind us that we are all a part of something much larger than ourselves. However you want to conceptualize it, looking up and out, being still, being present to what surrounds you, and making some space for wonder and reflection will almost surely help you put your problems in some manageable perspective.

I recently climbed Snowdon in Wales with a whole bunch of people. It was one of the most spiritually enjoyable days I have experienced in a while. The scenery was outstanding, and it got more amazing the higher we got. The air was thick and misty at the top of the mountain, and I took a few minutes to slip away from the party and sit by myself and enjoy that view. I felt as though my heart was expanding as I breathed in the cool mountain air and allowed time to stand still. It felt like a moment of surrender. I felt connected, renewed, and invigorated. I encourage you to connect with something that means something to you—it can be God, nature, or something else. We are all different, and our higher powers may vary. Yours could be music, art, or the family environment. There are no hard and fast rules here. Whatever it is, give yourself up to it and allow that connection to fill your heart, support you, and bring you peace.

During The Program, you want to make an effort to remind yourself that you are not alone. Get outside. Consider ways of exploring your own beliefs and strengthening your ties to whatever gives you comfort and makes you feel elevated, calm, supported, and connected to something greater than yourself, however that makes sense for you.

FRIENDS AND ACCOUNTABILITY PARTNERS

When you are healthier and feeling good, you are going to have more energy and self-confidence, and this often translates into healthier relationships with other people in your life. While you are getting there, you need people, preferably a whole network of people, who can support you while you pursue your goals.

At an absolute minimum, you need one person who can serve as an accountability partner. This is a person with whom you can be honest about your goals, to whom you can be vulnerable, who understands what you want and can help you get there. In an ideal world, this is a person you can train with, who can encourage you and maybe whom you can encourage as well. Your accountability partner can be someone who is in a similar position to you and can relate to your struggle, or it can be someone who is in outstanding and inspirational shape. The type of person who works best really varies for each individual. Think about what you need most. Will it be support in the gym? Will it be emotional support? Identify a person who you can trust to be reasonably available for you to check in with, who will help you through this process.

Sometimes people have a hard time visualizing their family members serving as accountability partners or being sources of support. If this is you, I encourage you to not write anyone off, because people can surprise you and it's a big help when your partner and family can get on board. But if yours won't, or they're far away, or they're not going to be able to fill this function for you for whatever reason, know that family comes in many different forms, and support for a healthy lifestyle doesn't have to come from your blood relatives. You can connect to a healthy network of people who are doing what you're doing and can encourage you. I have that at my gym. It's a place for me to connect with people as well as train, and it has a kind of family feeling for me. Most communities have resources of this kind, and they don't have to be expensive. Look into gyms, including your local YMCA and recreation department; biking, walking, and running groups and events; weight loss groups; and other organized exercise opportunities in your area. Walk through your local park and see if you see boot camps, yoga classes, or fitness equipment—identify things that indicate potentially appealing places for you to connect with other people who are doing what you're doing.

You also have online options for making fitness connections, including mine! Now that you've bought this book, you are part of The Program family. The Pavelka House is an online resource that provides you with a wealth of information and inspiration to keep you motivated and updated as well as being a great platform for linking up with other like-minded people. When I helped to design it, I wanted to create something that enhanced people's lives and helped keep them accountable, but didn't become a second job to keep it updated. I called it the House because it's somewhere you can check in to and feel part of something on your own terms.

The House is there when you need motivation or when you want to get ideas, record progress or celebrate with friends. People can have their own personal room in the House, too. Like with any room, you can decorate it when you move in. It's a place to keep pictures that make you feel inspired. No one else sees your room, so you can be as personal as you like. If you like a particular recipe, workout exercise, motivational quote, or story, you can click and save it to your room, then take it out again when you're ready to move on.

Community is an important part of The Program, and the forums and ability to comment on all of the articles in the House create conversation and interest among members, who learn from and encourage each other. One of my favorite parts of the House is the section where you can upload the events that you have set yourself as challenges. If you enter a 5K or a triathlon, you can upload the details and others who are in the area can get in touch and compare notes or meet up with you for training or the event itself. It's great fun, and I love seeing the public pictures members upload afterward!

The House is used differently by everyone. Some dip in and out for recipe ideas and workout suggestions, and maybe pop into the forums. Others are on there each day, and it has become part of their daily Program planning. The journal function means that you can capture your progress, feelings, and ideas. You are also able to set your monthly goals, and you will receive an email checking in with you each month so you are reminded to update or change them.

All of these functions help you to stay on track with The Program after reading the book, and I hope you'll check it out. (You can connect through JessiePavelka.com.) Online accountability partners can be very effective. I have clients who check in daily by text or email with people they've never met, but a "Did you work out today?" or "How are things going?" message keeps them motivated. Responsible online forums and communities can also be good resources for information about exercise and nutrition. These are helpful for anyone, and sometimes they are your only option for geographic or logistical reasons. But if you find that you are limiting yourself to online support because you are too intimidated to walk into a physical gym or connect with people in person, I encourage you to make doing that one of your subgoals as you get more comfortable following The Program. There are a lot of benefits to exercising with a partner or a group, which you can read about in more detail in the "Sweat" section of this book. Connecting with others is one of them.

By the way, kids can be great at making you accountable. If you've promised to take them somewhere (swimming, to the park or any physical activity) they will not let you off the hook. Trust me, I know this: my 6-year-old certainly keeps me on my toes. If you share your fitness goals or commitments with your kids, you might find that they are relentless in keeping you accountable and, possibly, thrilled to join you in some of your activities. You know yours best.

One other thing about connecting with others. In the same way that I want you to pay some mind to how you are thinking about and talking to yourself, pay attention to the quality of your communication with your family and friends. Take a minute to be conscious of your patterns when you interact. Do you look at one another? Is anyone checking the phone or multitasking while you're together? Are you checking your email when you're speaking on the phone? Are people listening or interrupting each other? Is your mind wandering when the other person is talking? I'm not judging, and you shouldn't either. Every conversation we have isn't going to be a meaningful and reflective one. But notice what has become normal for you, and think about making an effort to improve the quality of the connections you have with the people you care about.

COMMUNITY

I've noticed that my unhappy clients have tended to withdraw from the world. It's understandable that when we don't feel good, it's harder to feel positive or interested in engaging with others. I worked with a young guy, Ben, who had been overweight all his life and had experienced bullying and teasing as a boy to the extent that he just assumed everyone was judging him negatively. He withdrew as an adult as a way of protecting himself and had become almost socially paralyzed. Now, you may not be in such an extreme situation. But you might be unhappy with how you look, less socially confident than you wish you were, or maybe even just lonely. If this is you, I get the impulse to isolate when you are unhappy. I have been there, and I know that it only prolongs and intensifies your suffering. The worse you feel, whether it's about your weight or something else, the more important it is for you to be connected with people who care about you and the wider world.

When you consider your current network of people to identify an accountability partner, you may also be able to see different sources of potential support from different people. Maybe there's one person who will work out with you on a more casual basis. Maybe there is someone else who can help you make time to fit exercise into your life, like a coworker who might be interested in walking together on your lunch break or a friend who might be willing to watch your kids for an hour while you work out. Is there someone who might share an interest in talking with you about healthy food and cooking? How about people who are just going to care about you and listen when you're frustrated and celebrate your success? Every kind of support you are able to harness is going to help you, and you may find that your decisions inspire and support other people to make healthy changes in their lives as well. You just need to be brave enough to put your goals out there and enlist that help.

If you don't think you have those people, I am challenging you to find them by engaging in your community. Take a fitness class, sign up for an event, consider volunteering—anything that can help expand your network to include other people who are also making healthy choices and can help you stay motivated, encouraged, and inspired. There is power in groups, in healthy competition, and in being stimulated by new experiences. Tapping into any of that will enhance your experience on The Program.

I have noticed a really cool thing happening with a group of my clients. I always encourage people to set individual challenges (for example, to run a 5K) to get them excited about their new way of life and give them something to aim for. What is happening more and more is that groups of my clients are coming together to train, practice, and take part in a variety of different events and occasions. Mud runs, zip wires, spa weekends, charity runs, you name it: they are constantly surprising me with the ways they are finding to unite as a community through fitness. Their enthusiasm and energy is inspiring. Look for ways that you can bring people together. You don't have to wait for someone else to organize something, you can be a leader, a pioneer. You will bring joy and health to others and feel amazing.

A Word about Problem People

Some of my clients discover that one or more people they are connected with are not so supportive of their efforts to be healthy. It's very common, and you do need to deal with it. If you notice that your partner keeps bringing home your favorite cookies from the bakery or throws up a lot of obstacles when you are scheduling your workouts, or that your mom gets offended if you don't come back for seconds at her dinner table, try to connect with those people in a calm, nonjudgmental way and talk about what's happening. Say something like, "I'm noticing [this] and it makes it hard for me to do [that]." See what they say. Sometimes well-meaning people don't understand your goals or didn't realize how their behavior is interfering with your efforts to get healthy. You can usually figure that out together. Other times, it's more complicated. If you find that there are people in your life who can't or won't change on issues that interfere with your taking care of yourself, you need set some boundaries.

Setting healthy boundaries doesn't necessarily mean cutting off a relationship. Depending on the situation, you might not even have to tell someone you're doing it. But if you are attached to people who make it hard for you to stick with The Program, you need to sort out ways to interact with them that don't involve unhealthy food, don't interfere with your exercise, and don't make you feel bad about yourself, depending on the situation. Sometimes this is as simple as suggesting meeting a friend over a coffee or morning walk instead of dinner or evening drinks at a bar. Sometimes it's more complicated—and disappointing—to discover that someone you want to rely on is not going to be able to support you in this way. Developing and maintaining a wider network of healthy relationships will go a long way toward helping you navigate this.

WORKING ON RELATIONSHIPS

The stronger all of these relationships in your life are, the better you're going to feel and the more likely you are to achieve success on The Program, however you are defining it. Cultivating these connections will take time, patience, and some trial and error. Make it a priority to take one action each day to connect on one of these relationships during The Program. Put it on your to-do list if you have to, and notice if you tend to be cultivating one or two types of relationships at the expense of all four. Try to spread your energy around a bit and plant seeds in all four areas over the course of each week, and look forward to seeing what blooms.

The Rest of Your Life

Changing your body is also about changing your mind. There are a bunch of different ways to get results in a mirror or on a scale, but the key to living well over the long term is developing the ability to take care of yourself no matter what else is happening in your life. I hope that you'll use The Program to Eat, Sweat, Think, and Connect your way to the very best version of yourself.

Once you complete the first cycle of The Program, take some time to reflect. Repeat the fitness assessments and evaluate your progress. Appreciate your amazing body and what it can do. Identify what parts of The Program are going well and what is still challenging. Troubleshoot those challenges. Is your goal realistic? Are you making it a priority? Have you learned or improved anything during the process of chasing it, even if you have not reached it yet?

Be realistic. There are parts of your body that can be changed and parts that genetically belong to you. Understand the difference between them, and don't waste time agonizing about stuff that isn't under your control. Look at all the different types of athletic body shapes, notice how different they are, and how few of them are what we might call skinny. Seek out body images and messages that reflect health and reinforce the power of good performance. You can control a lot: be consistent about your workouts, give them your all, and fuel them properly. Focus on your effort. Don't only notice how you look. Notice how you feel.

I don't know you, and I don't know what your goals are. But I hope, at this point in The Program, that they aren't just about getting thin. Our bodies come in all shapes and sizes. Being strong is sexy. Being fit is powerful. Being confident is beautiful. Living well is inspiring. Being healthy frees up energy in your life to pursue the things and relationships that make you feel good. You can be all those things and look amazing and not be skinny. I hope you are thinking about yourself as an athlete, and that you understand the power that nutrition, rest, and commitment have on your ability to perform at your best. I hope that you are becoming more aware of your unique gifts and potential, and are making richer connections with others that help support you in reaching your goals and enhancing your life.

You may be humbled and challenged at points on The Program, but I hope you're also getting to feel fully present and alive, and experiencing the satisfaction that comes from taking good care of yourself and pushing to be your very best. That may be stronger, slimmer, and sexier, but it's fundamentally about living well.

Training Schedule

Day	Program
1	Strength assessment
2	Athletic assessment
3	Metabolic assessment
4	Slow burn and flow assessment
5	Metabolic training
6	Strength training
7	Athletic training
8	Strength training
9	Metabolic training
10	Strength training
11	Athletic training
12	Strength training
13	Slow burn and flow

Day	Program
14	Strength training
15	Athletic training
16	Strength training
17	Metabolic training
18	Strength training
19	Athletic training
20	Strength training
21	Metabolic training
22	Choose your training
23	Retest starts
EXTRAS	Weekend Warrior
	Yoga

The Program Workouts

The Program workouts are divided by level: beginner ("Getting Started"), intermediate ("Ramp It Up"), and advanced ("Full Throttle"). As with all other areas of The Program, I want this to be as flexible as possible so that it works for you. If you need to follow the Getting Started workouts for the strength workouts but are ready to do Ramp It Up for your burn-agility workouts, feel free to flip around. Also, I want you to be able to use these training plans for as long as possible! If you're improving when you repeat the assessment tests, take it to the next level workout and see how it feels.

The tests should all take you less than 20 minutes, including time spent sorting out the exercises. Review the moves and maybe do a practice or two to make sure you've got it down. Then get a wristwatch or phone with a timer handy, perform each one on the clock, and record the results.

DON'T SKIP THE WARM-UP!

Whenever you are exercising, it's helpful to prime the body for movement. Spend about a minute doing each of the following movements before you get started with any of the workouts and assessments on The Program. You don't have to worry about levels here. Everyone can warm up in the same way.

Repeat each exercise for 30–45 seconds:

Squat (see page 57 for photos)

Setup: Stand with your feet hip-width apart, arms at your sides.

Action: Bend your knees like you're sitting in a chair until your thighs are nearly parallel to the floor. Slowly return to start position.

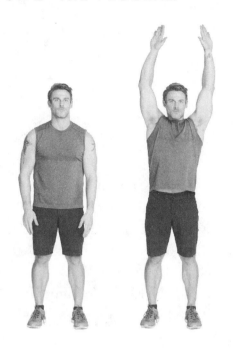

Arm Circle

Setup: Start standing with feet shoulder-width apart, arms at your sides.

Action: Slowly start to make circles of about 1 foot in diameter with your arms. Continue 10 times, then change direction.

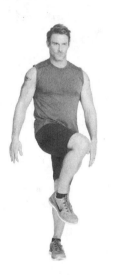
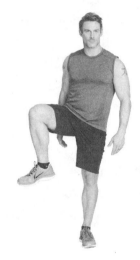

Hip Opener

Setup: Stand with your feet hip-width apart.

Raise your right knee up toward your chest and rotate it to the right in a circular motion, lower it, and repeat 10 times on each side.

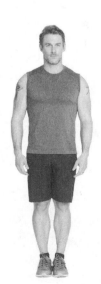
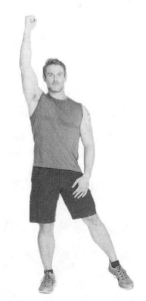

Half Jack

Setup: Start standing with your arms by your sides.

Action: Tap your right leg out to your right side as you reach your left arm up to the ceiling. Repeat on the other side.

DAY 1: FITNESS ASSESSMENT (ALL LEVELS) AND SLOW BURN CARDIO

Strength

You will need a stopwatch, a mat, and a bench or sturdy chair. You will also need a pen and paper to record your repetitions and time held.

Perform each exercise for 30 seconds (except Plank, which you will hold for as long as you can while timing yourself), count each repetition as you do it, then write it down and rest for 60 seconds before moving on to the next exercise.

Once you have recorded all exercises, total the number and divide by 4. This will determine the level of exercise you should start at.

Getting Started: 0–29
Ramp It Up: 30–35
Full Throttle: 35+

For example, you do:

Push-up: 15 reps
Plank: Held for 65 seconds
Squat: 12 reps
Triceps Dip: 16 reps
Total: 108

Divide the total number by 4 to get 27. This person will perform the Getting Started strength workouts.

DAY 1, PART 1: INSTRUCTIONS FOR STRENGTH EXERCISES

■ Push-up

Setup: Start on the floor lying on your stomach, with your hands close to your chest and your elbows at a 45-degree angle.

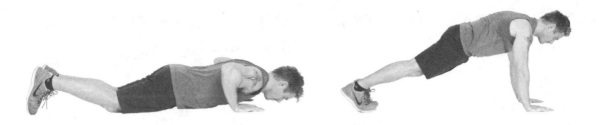

Action: Raise yourself off the floor until your arms are fully extended. Your hands and the balls of your feet should support your weight. Keep a straight line from your head to your heels, contracting your abdominals and glutes so your hips don't sag. Lower your chest to the floor. Repeat.

✱ *If performing push-ups on your knees, subtract 5 from total number of push-ups.*

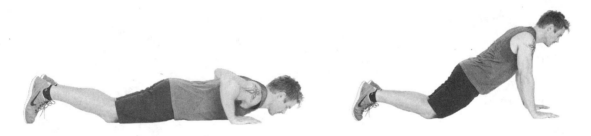

■ Squat (see page 57 for photos)

Setup: Stand with your feet hip-width apart, arms at your sides.

Action: Bend your knees like you're sitting in a chair until your thighs are nearly parallel to the floor. Slowly return to start position.

■ Plank

Setup: Get into a push-up position, bend your elbows, and bring your weight to your forearms instead of your hands.

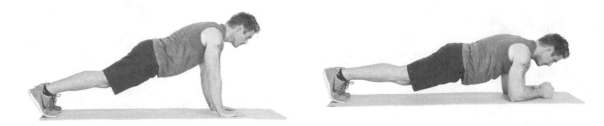

Action: Brace your abdominal muscles and keep a straight line from your shoulders to your ankles. Record how long you can hold a plank with good form. If performing a plank on your knees, subtract 15 from total number of seconds held.

■ Triceps Dip

Setup: Sit on the edge of bench or sturdy chair, hands grasping the seat on either side of your hips. Keep your feet flat on the floor with your knees bent, and bring your hips off the edge of the bench or chair.

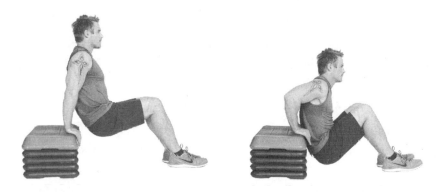

Action: Bend your elbows and lower your hips toward the floor. Straighten your arms and return to starting position.

DAY 1, PART 2: GET IN MOTION

You'll be moving more than you used to on The Program. During the first four Cleanse days, while you're eating pretty lightly, you'll do about 20 minutes of light cardio exercise in addition to the daily fitness assessments. After the first 4 days of The Program, you'll be doing a more intense Wake-Up Workout each morning and a workout routine associated with one of the assessed fitness areas every day, but you can also challenge yourself to continue to walk or run on any or all of the remaining Program days. Many people find they really enjoy it. For today, it's just the assessment and the walk or run. There's no test for this one. I'm relying on you to give yourself a reasonable challenge if you choose to take it. Do the warm-up, then spend 20 minutes in motion today in one of the following ways.

Beginner: If you have been completely or primarily sedentary before beginning The Program, set aside 20 minutes to walk. Don't worry about how far or fast you go during that time. The point is to just get back into motion and see how you feel. Our bodies were made to walk, and you don't require any training background to do it. Just put on a comfortable pair of shoes and get outside. Think about the weather and try to go at a time of day when it won't be extreme. Bring some water with you if you think you'll need it. Enjoy your walk, and slow down or rest if you feel breathless.

Intermediate: If you feel like walking for 20 minutes would be no big deal for you, try walking that amount of time briskly. If you have a timer or step tracker on your phone or wristwatch, try using it and see if you can't cover a mile and a half in 20 minutes. Walking a mile in about 15 minutes is a brisk pace. You shouldn't be feeling overwhelmed, but you'll get a bit more of a workout and start recruiting a higher percentage of your slow twitch muscle fibers.

Advanced: You can spend your 20 minutes alternating walking with jogging at a very comfortable pace. Start by walking for a few minutes, then jog at a pace such that you could still have a conversation with someone. When you feel like you're working too hard to do that, or even if you're just noticing that you're breathing heavily, slow down to a walk and keep walking until you feel completely recovered. Pick up the jog again when you feel ready. You might alternate between walking and jogging four times each in 20 minutes, or even 10 times, whatever is comfortable for you.

Expert: If you are already pretty fit, jog continuously for 20 minutes each day during the Cleanse portion of The Program. You are not sprinting, so don't worry about your pace at all. You just want a comfortable, easy jog on relatively flat ground. If you feel breathless after 10 or 15 minutes, slow down to a brisk walk until you are completely recovered, then resume jogging.

Whatever you decide to do, if you feel spent, breathless, and exhausted at the end of your 20 minutes, go down a level tomorrow. The point here is to be in motion, not push it to the max. The feeling you're going for is to be energized and refreshed after some mild activity, and perhaps to be excited to do it again tomorrow. You should ideally feel like you could have kept going for another 10 minutes, because after 4 days of this you'll be primed for more intense exercise.

DAY 2: FITNESS ASSESSMENT (ALL LEVELS)

Athletic

You will need a stopwatch and a clear area of space to move in (ideally not carpeted). You will also need a pen and paper to record your repetitions.

Perform each exercise for 30 seconds, count each repetition as you do it, then write it down and rest for 60 seconds before moving on to the next exercise. Once you have recorded all exercises, total the number and divide by 4. This will determine the level of exercise you should start at.

Getting Started: 0–24
Ramp It Up: 25–34
Full Throttle: 35+

For example, if you do:

Side Shuffle Tap: 25
Jump Rope: 35
Pass the Ball, Shoot the Ball: 17
Speed Skate: 27
Total: 104

Divide the total number by 4 to get 26. This person will do the Ramp It Up athletic workouts.

DAY 2, PART 1: INSTRUCTIONS FOR ATHLETIC EXERCISES

■ Side Shuffle

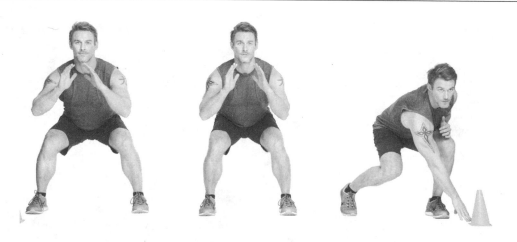

Setup: Stand with your feet shoulder-width apart, knees slightly bent.

Action: Take a large step out to your right with your right foot, bring your left foot over to meet the right, take another large step to the right with your right foot, then bend your knees and tap the floor with your left hand. Repeat in the other direction. Count one repetition for each tap.

▪ Jump Rope Right/Left

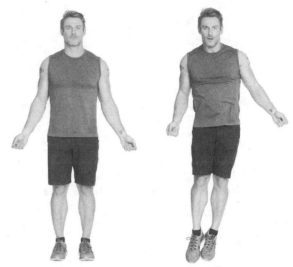

Setup: Stand with your feet together and imagine you are holding jump rope handles.

Action: Push off the floor with the balls of your feet, and jump softly to your right. Push off again, and jump softly to your left.

▪ Pass the Ball, Shoot the Ball

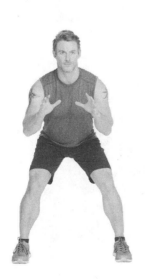
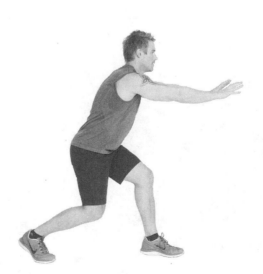
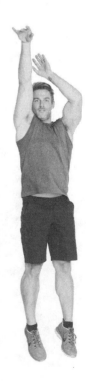

Setup: Stand with your feet slightly wider than hip-width apart, knees slightly bent and hands at chest level.

Action: Imagine you are holding a basketball at your chest. Pivot to your right side and push your arms out as if passing the ball. Come back to starting position and jump up or lift up on your toes and pretend to shoot the ball. One rep is counted for each time you shoot the ball. If you are lifting on your toes instead of jumping, subtract 10 from the total number of repetitions.

■ Speed Skate

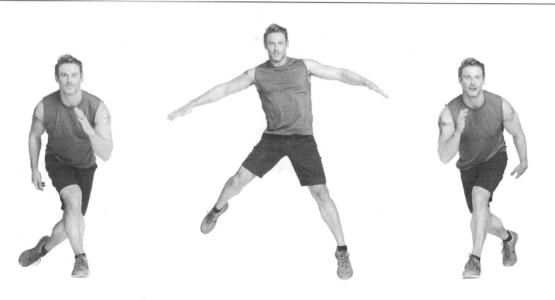

Setup: Stand with your feet hip-width apart, knees slightly bent.

Action: Leap or step to the right side and land on your right leg, reaching down with your right hand toward your right knee or toes. Leap or step to the left side and land on your left leg, reaching down with your left hand toward your left knee or toes.

DAY 2, PART 2:

Walk or jog for 20 minutes, following the instructions from day 1. If you were very tired after what you did yesterday, go down a level. If you feel like you could have gone harder, feel free to try the next level up. Remember, the point is to just to enjoy being in motion today, not to push it really hard. If you are sore, go down a level or walk for a shorter distance, but don't skip this exercise. The kind of walking I'm asking you to do is good for sore muscles and will make you feel better than simply resting.

DAY 3: FITNESS ASSESSMENT (ALL LEVELS)

Metabolic

You will need a stopwatch and a sturdy wall to lean against. You will also need a pen and paper to record your repetitions and time held.

Perform each exercise for 30 seconds (except for the Wall Sit, which is for time held), count each repetition as you do it, then write it down and rest for 60 seconds before moving on to the next exercise.

Once you have recorded all exercises, total the number and divide by 4. This will determine the level of exercise you should start at.

Getting Started: 0–30
Ramp It Up: 30–50
Full Throttle: 50+

For example, if you do:

Squat Thrust: 15
High Knee: 43
Wall Sit: Held for 110 seconds
Alternating Lateral Lunge: 18
Total: 186

Divide the total number by 4 to get 46. This person will do the Ramp It Up metabolic workouts.

DAY 3, PART 1: INSTRUCTIONS FOR METABOLIC EXERCISES

■ Squat Thrust

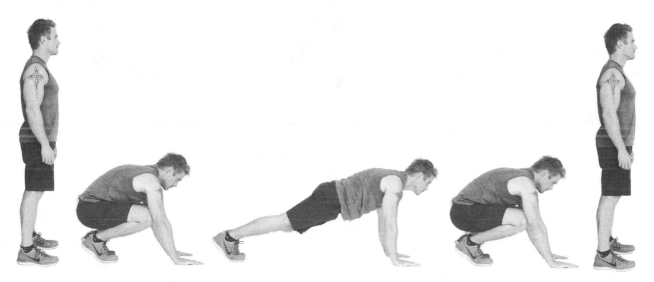

Setup: Stand with your feet together, arms at your sides.

Action: Bend your knees and place your palms on the floor with your arms on the outside of your knees. Shift your weight onto your palms. Jump both feet back and land in plank position or walk one foot at a time into plank position. Jump both feet forward and return to standing. If you are stepping into plank position, subtract 5 from the total number of repetitions.

■ High Knee

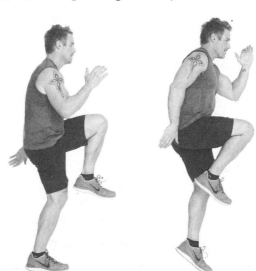

Setup: Stand with feet hip-width apart, knees slightly bent, and elbows bent 90 degrees.

Action: Bring your right knee up to hip level, push off your left foot, and switch legs, bringing your left leg up to hip level. Continue running in place and touching your hand to your thighs each time your leg comes up.

■ Alternating Lateral Lunge

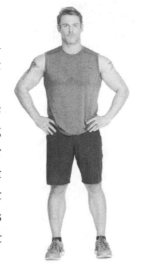
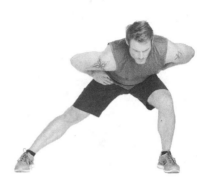

Setup: Stand with your feet together, hands on your hips.

Action: Take a big step to the right, keeping your left toes pointing straight ahead, and bending your right knee until your thigh is almost parallel to the floor. Keep your left knee straight but not locked. Press off your right foot to return to start position. Repeat on other leg.

■ Wall Sit

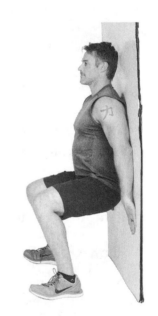

Setup: Stand with your back against a wall, placing your feet about 2 feet in front of you. Your feet should be hip-width apart.

Action: Bend your knees, and slide down the wall until your knees are at 90-degree angles. Your knees should be over your ankles, and your thighs should be parallel. Place your palms on the wall.

DAY 3, PART 2:

Walk or jog for 20 minutes, following the instructions from day 2.

DAY 4: FITNESS ASSESSMENT (ALL LEVELS)

Slow Burn and Flow

DAY 4, PART 1:

This slow burn exercise is to assess your current aerobic endurance. You will need an outdoor area where you can walk, jog, or run, or access to a treadmill. This is a little different than the way I asked you to walk or jog over the last 3 days (you'll still need to do that today as well), because I want you to record the distance you cover in 10 minutes. If you want to continue walking or jogging for 10 additional minutes and call that your slow burn cardio for the day, you can, or you can take this test and then go for a 20-minute walk or jog without worrying about timing anything later in the day. It's up to you.

Setup: Begin with a 3-minute walk at a comfortable pace.

Action: Walk, jog, or run for 10 minutes. Record the distance. For example, you might record two laps around a standard track, or ½ mile, in 10 minutes. There are many applications you can download on your phone to do this for you if you don't have a good sense of the distance on your own.

The distance you cover determines your level of fitness at steady-state cardio activity. If you record two laps around a standard track, or ½ mile, in 10 minutes, you should do the Ramp It Up level of the slow burn and flow workout. (See page 148 for the Ramp It Up level of the slow burn and flow workout.)

The flow is a series of five yoga postures for increased range of motion: Downward-Facing Dog, Warrior I, Warrior II, Side Angle, and Child's Pose. These poses focus on stretching the major muscle groups you will be using during your workouts (chest, shoulders, thighs, hip flexors, and back). You are not scoring yourself on these poses; you just want to learn how to do them, see how they feel, then use this series as a cool-down after your regular workouts, or at any point that you want to work on increasing your flexibility and range of motion.

✳ *You will need a yoga mat.*

DAY 4, PART 2: INSTRUCTIONS FOR FLOW EXERCISES

■ Downward-Facing Dog

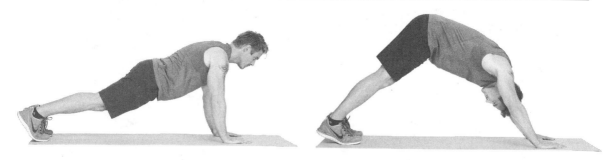

Setup: Begin in a plank position. As you inhale, spread your fingers wide and press both palms firmly into the mat while simultaneously tucking your toes under. As you exhale, begin to draw your hips toward the ceiling, making the shape of an inverted V. Your head and neck should be between your upper arms. Bend your knees as much as you need to while maintaining equal weight on your hands and feet. Hold for three to five breath cycles.

Flow from Downward-Facing Dog into Low Lunge.

■ Low Lunge

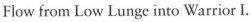

Step your right foot between your hands, coming into a low lunge position. Shift your weight forward slightly to allow your right thigh to become parallel to the floor while remaining on the ball of your back foot (that should be your left foot).

Flow from Low Lunge into Warrior I.

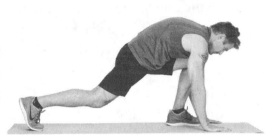

■ Warrior I

Keeping your front foot facing forward, turn your back foot slightly outward and let your back foot rest flat at a 45-degree angle. Reach your arms overhead so they are parallel to one another. Your hips should still be facing forward as you lower your shoulders away from your ears and lift your core as you bend your front knee (your right knee) into a 90-degree angle. Hold this position for three to five breath cycles.

Flow from Warrior I into Warrior II.

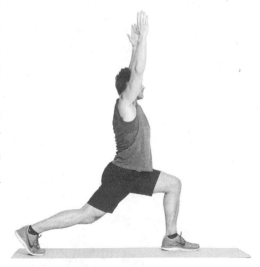

■ Warrior II

Rotate your weight to the left and bring your arms straight out to your sides, parallel to the floor. Although the position of your feet does not change, your hips should now face the left. Your front leg (your right leg) should be bent while your back (left leg) is straight. This is Warrior II pose. Hold it for three to five breath cycles.

Flow from Warrior II into Side Angle.

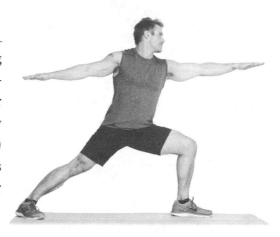

■ Side Angle

Drop your right forearm on your right thigh and tilt your torso open, so that your left hand is now up in the air, reaching for the ceiling. Hold for three to five breath cycles.

Repeat this sequence on the other side. This means that you'll step back with your right leg back into Downward-Facing Dog and repeat the entire flow on your left side.

Continue to alternate sets between sides two to five times.

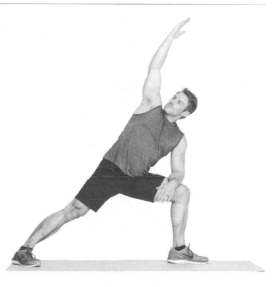

DAY 4, PART 3:

If you did not extend the Slow Burn Assessment test to walk or jog for 10 additional minutes, make sure you still do a 20-minute walk or jog today, following the instructions from day 1. Feel free to mix it up by going down or up a level depending on how you feel, and remember that the point is to enjoy being in motion. You'll start the leveled workouts tomorrow, so don't overdo it!

BONUS WORKOUT: 5 CORE STRENGTH EXERCISES

Many of my clients want to focus on their core strength or to target weight loss in that area. There are many ways of moving that strengthen the core, and everything you're doing in the workouts during The Program will help you lose weight. But if you're interested in doing some extra moves, consider adding these to your routine or fitting in this little workout in the same way you might make time for a quick stretch workout if you're working on flexibility.

Getting Started: Perform 10 reps of each exercise, rest for 30 seconds, then move on to the next exercise. Repeat the circuit three times.

Ramp It Up: Perform 20 reps of each exercise, rest for 30 seconds, then move on to the next exercise. Repeat the circuit three times.

Full Throttle: Perform 30 reps of each exercise, rest for 30 seconds, then move on to the next exercise. Repeat the circuit three times.

Between each set perform eight back extensions (instructions below).

■ Crunch

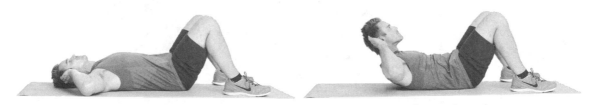

Setup: Lie faceup with your knees bent, feet flat on the floor, and hands behind your head with fingertips lightly touching.

Action: Lift your shoulders off the floor until you feel a tight contraction on your abdominals. Return to starting position and repeat.

■ Reverse Crunch

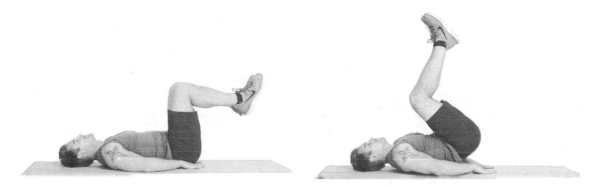

Setup: Lie faceup on the floor. Place both hands by your hips, palms down.

Action: Keeping your knees and ankles together, bring your knees toward your chest. Squeeze your abdominals to lift your hips and legs toward the ceiling.

Lower your legs and repeat.

* *Jessie's Tip: Don't use your legs as momentum to lift up. Focus on the power coming from your abs.*

■ Stability Ball Crunch

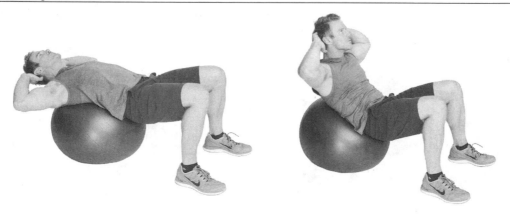

Setup: Sit on the ball, walk forward, and rest your low back on the ball. Bend your knees and keep your feet flat on the floor. Place your hands behind your head.

Action: Contract your abdominals to lift your torso off the ball, drawing your belly button toward your spine. Return to start position.

▪ Stability Ball Oblique Crunch

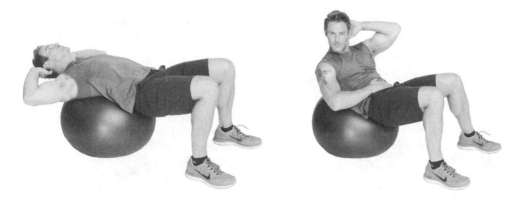

Setup: Sit on the ball, walk forward, and rest your low back on the ball. Bend your knees and keep your feet flat on the floor. Place your right hand behind your head and your left hand at your navel.

Action: Contract your abdominals to lift your torso off the ball, and twist over toward your left knee, drawing your belly button toward your spine. Return to start position. Repeat all reps, then change sides.

▪ Stability Ball Pike

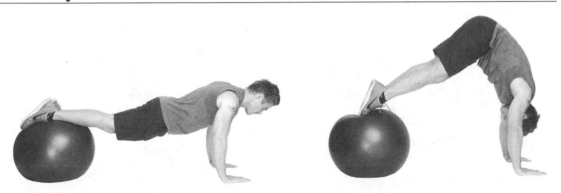

Setup: Start with your torso on the ball and hands and feet on the floor. Walk your hands forward until your ankles are on top of the ball.

Action: Keeping your legs straight, pull your feet toward your chest, raise your hips toward the ceiling as the ball rolls in, and continue until your hips are directly under your shoulders. Slowly lower back to starting position.

✳ *Jessie's Tip: To make it less challenging, keep your knees bent.*

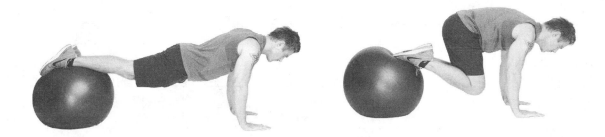

Between each set perform eight back extensions (instructions below).

■ Stability Ball Back Extension

Setup: Lie facedown on a stability ball with your hands on the ball at your sides,

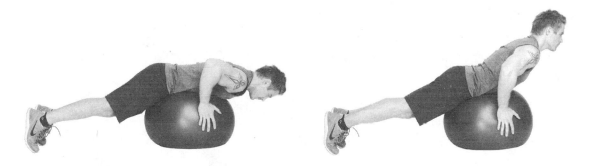

about 6 inches apart. Press your feet against a wall or sturdy object.

Action: Lift your torso up until your body forms a straight line.

* *Jessie's Tip: To make it more challenging, perform the exercise with your fingertips by your ears instead of on the ball.*

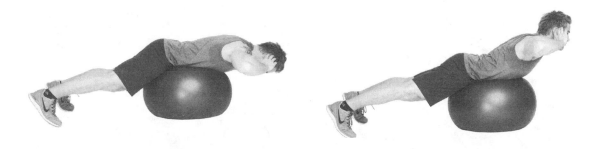

GETTING STARTED (BEGINNER)

Wake-up Workout

Getting Started	Ramp It Up	Full Throttle
Jumping Jacks or Half Jacks	Jumping Jacks	Jumping Jacks
Squats	Push-ups	Squat Thrusts
Knee Push-ups	Lateral Lunges	Push-ups
Alternating Lunges	Plank with Alternating Knee Cross	Split Lunge Jumps

GETTING STARTED WAKE-UP WORKOUT

This 4-minute circuit will get you ready and energized for a healthy day. You'll start each morning from day 5 of The Program onward with this workout. You will be doing each exercise for 20 seconds, recovering for 10 seconds, then moving on to the next exercise. Repeat the circuit two times.

■ Jumping Jack

Setup: Start standing with your arms by your sides.

Action: Jump your legs out to the sides as you bring your arms overhead.

Jump your feet back together and return arms to your sides.

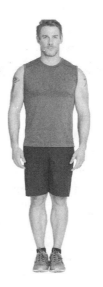
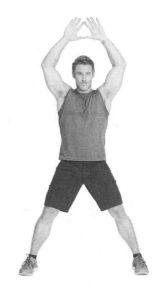

■ Half Jack

Setup: Start standing with your arms by your sides.

Action: Tap your right leg out to your right side as you reach your left arm up to the ceiling. Repeat on the other side.

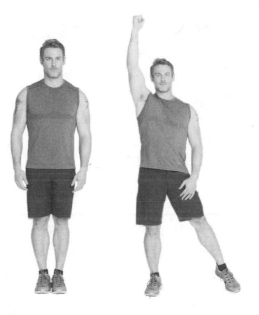

■ Squat (see page 57 for photos)

Setup: Stand with your feet hip-width apart, arms at your sides.

Action: Bend your knees like you're sitting in a chair until your thighs are nearly parallel to the floor. Slowly return to start position.

■ Knee Push-up (see page 86 for photos)

Setup: Start on your hands and knees. Straighten your torso and place your hands directly underneath your shoulders, slightly wider than your shoulders, and rest on your knees.

Action: Bend your elbows and slowly lower your chest toward the floor. Push up to start position.

▪ Reverse Lunge

Setup: Stand shoulder-width apart.

Action: Take a step backward with your right leg, lowering your right knee toward the floor. Push off the right foot to come back to start position. Repeat, alternating legs.

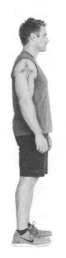
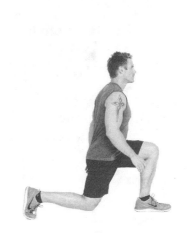

GETTING STARTED DAY 5: BURN—METABOLIC TRAINING

Perform each exercise for 60 seconds, then move on to the next exercise. Complete one circuit, recover for 90 seconds, then repeat the circuit five times.

▪ Squat with Dumbbell Overhead Press

Setup: Stand with your feet hip-width apart, holding a dumbbell in each hand at your shoulders, palms facing in.

Action: Bend your knees like you're sitting in a chair until your thighs are nearly parallel to the floor. As you rise out of the squat, lift the dumbbells overhead until they are about an inch apart. Lower the dumbbells as you return to start position.

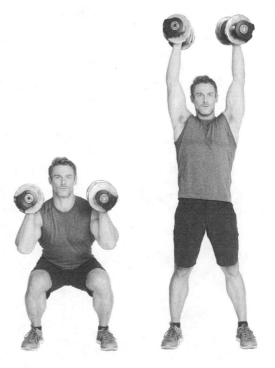

■ Alternating Step-up

Setup: Stand with your feet hip-width apart in front of a bench.

Action: Place your right foot on the bench so that your foot is completely on the bench. Push through your right heel to raise your body onto the bench, tap your left foot to the top of the bench, and return to starting position, then step up with your left foot. Continue, alternating legs.

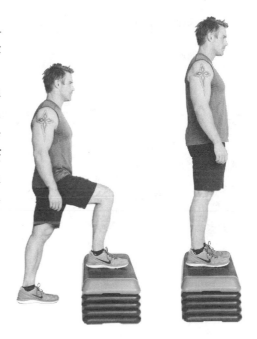

■ Sumo Squat Biceps Curl

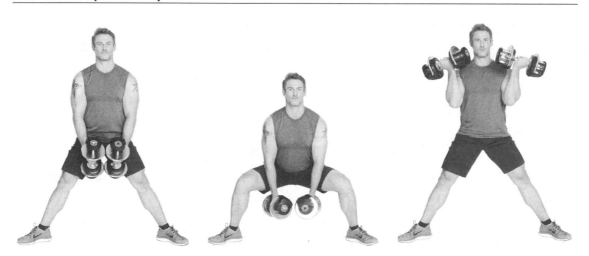

Setup: Stand with your feet slightly wider than hip-width apart, toes out, arms in front of you, holding a dumbbell in each hand, palms facing inward.

Action: Bend your knees and lower your body until your thighs are parallel to the floor. Push yourself back up as you rotate your wrists outward and curl the dumbbells to your shoulders.

■ Reverse Lunge Lateral Raise

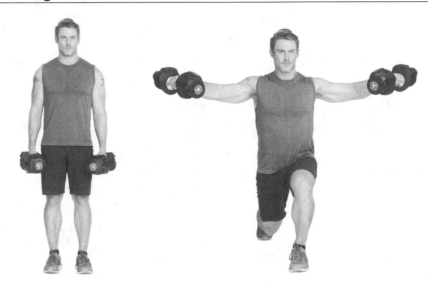

Setup: Stand with your feet shoulder-width apart with a dumbbell in each hand, arms down at your sides, palms facing each other.

Action: Take a step backward with your right leg, lowering your right knee toward the floor, simultaneously lifting the dumbbells out to the sides to shoulder level. Return to starting position. Continue, alternating legs.

■ Crunch (see page 98 for photos)

Setup: Lie faceup with your knees bent, feet flat on the floor, and hands behind your head with fingertips lightly touching.

Action: Lift your shoulders off the floor until you feel a tight contraction on your abdominals. Return to starting position and repeat.

GETTING STARTED DAY 6: BUILD—STRENGTH TRAINING

■ Push Day

Five sets of five reps
    Recovery: 30–60 seconds between sets

▪ Knee Push-up (see page 86 for photos)

Setup: Start on your hands and knees. Straighten your torso and place your hands directly underneath your shoulders, slightly wider than your shoulders, and rest on your knees.

Action: Bend your elbows and slowly lower your chest toward the floor. Push up to start position.

▪ Shoulder Press

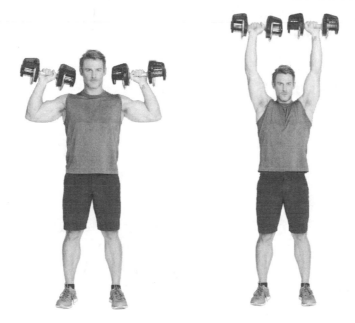

Setup: Stand with your feet shoulder-width apart, holding a dumbbell in each hand at shoulder level.

Action: Press the dumbbells overhead, keeping your arms in line with your ears. Slowly lower your arms to shoulder height.

▪ Triceps Dip (see page 87 for photos)

Setup: Sit on the edge of bench or sturdy chair, hands grasping the seat on either side of your hips. Keep your feet flat on the floor with your knees bent, and bring your hips off the edge of the bench or chair.

Action: Bend your elbows and lower your hips toward the floor. Straighten your arms and return to starting position.

◼ Lateral Raise

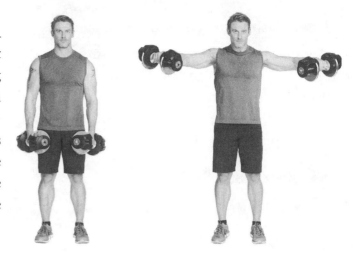

Setup: Stand with your feet shoulder-width apart, holding a dumbbell in each hand with palms facing in.

Action: Keeping your arms straight but not locked, raise the dumbbells out to the side in line with your shoulders. Lower the dumbbells to starting position.

◼ Dumbbell Chest Fly

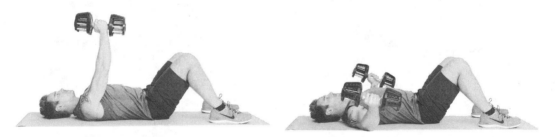

Setup: Lie back on an exercise bench or mat with a dumbbell in each hand, palms facing in. Extend the dumbbells over your chest.

Action: Lower your arms until the weights are even with your chest. Press the dumbbells back to starting position.

GETTING STARTED DAY 7: BURN—ATHLETIC TRAINING

◼ HIIT Athletic Training

Alternate 30 seconds of work and 30 seconds of recovery.

Do all four exercises 30 seconds on, then 30 seconds off, one after the other, then recover for 1 minute. Repeat the circuit four times.

■ Pass the Ball, Shoot the Ball (see page 90 for photos)

Setup: Stand with your feet slightly wider than hip-width apart, knees slightly bent and hands at chest level.

Action: Imagine you are holding a basketball at your chest. Pivot to your right side and push your arms out as if passing the ball. Come back to starting position and jump up or lift up on your toes and pretend to shoot the ball. Repeat on the other side.

■ Side Shuffle (see page 89 for photos)

Setup: Stand with your feet shoulder-width apart, knees slightly bent.

Action: Take a large step out to your right with your right foot, bring your left foot over to meet the right, take another large step to the right with your right foot, then bend your knees to tap the floor with your left hand. Repeat in the other direction.

■ Lunge Kick Lunge

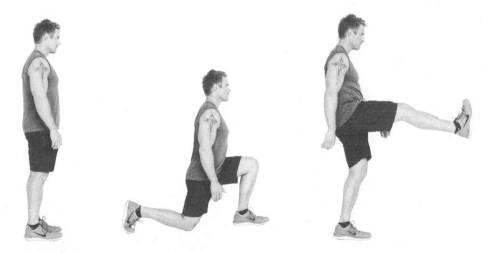

Setup: Stand with feet shoulder-width apart with knees slightly bent.

Action: Step back with your right foot into a lunge, press off the ball of your right foot, and kick your right leg forward.

Repeat for 30 seconds, switching sides on the next circuit.

✴ *Jessie's Tip: Don't worry about how high you kick. Focus on your balance and keeping your core engaged.*

■ Alternating Elbow to Knee

Setup: Stand with your feet shoulder-width apart and extend your right arm up and your left leg to the side.

Action: Lower your right elbow and raise your left knee, crunching them together on a diagonal line. Repeat for 30 seconds, switching sides on the next circuit.

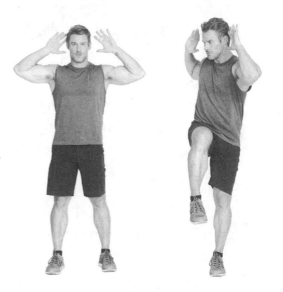

GETTING STARTED DAY 8: BUILD—STRENGTH

■ Pull Day

Five sets of five reps
Recovery: 30–60 seconds between sets

■ Dumbbell Row

Setup: Stand with your feet hip-width apart with a dumbbell in each hand, palms facing in. Hinge forward to a 45-degree angle from the hips, keeping your back long and knees slightly bent.

Action: Pull the dumbbells up until your elbows pass your torso. Lower to starting position.

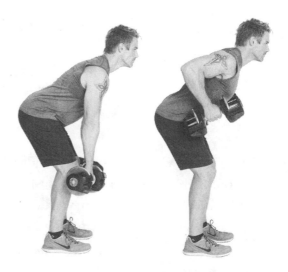

◼ **Biceps Curl**

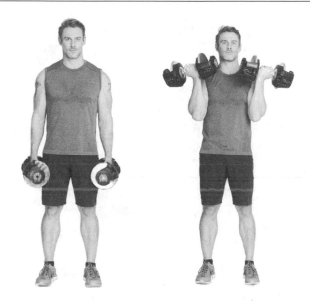

Setup: Stand with your feet hip-width apart holding a dumbbell in each hand, palms facing forward.

Action: Curl the weights toward your shoulders, then return to the starting position.

◼ **Lat Pullover**

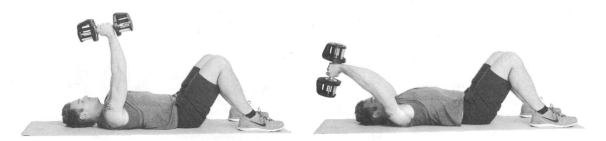

Setup: Lie faceup on a bench or mat. Hold a dumbbell in each hand over your chest, keeping your elbows slightly bent.

Action: Extend your arms over your chest, palms facing in. Keeping your elbows slightly bent, lower the dumbbells in an arc back over your head toward the floor. Bring your elbows level with your head, then return to start position.

■ Resistance Band Row

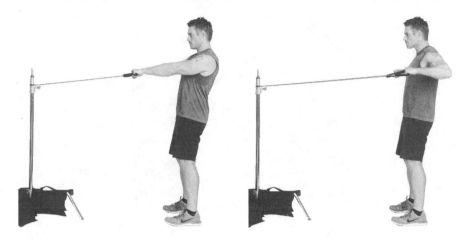

Setup: Attach the resistance band door attachment at chest height. Stand facing the door, holding both handles and with your knees slightly bent.

Action: Reach forward with your arms in line with your shoulders. Pull the band back until your elbows pass your torso. Return to start.

■ Back Extension with Alternating Arm Raise

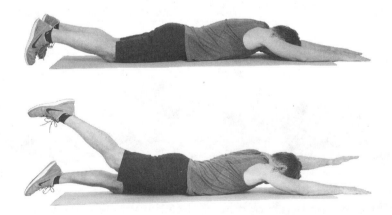

Setup: Lie facedown on a mat with your arms and legs extended.

Action: Keeping your neck in line with your spine, lift your right leg and left arm off the mat. Return to start, and repeat on the other side.

GETTING STARTED DAY 9: BURN—METABOLIC TRAINING

■ Five Exercises, 1 Minute Each Exercise, Repeat Circuit Three Times

Perform each exercise for 60 seconds, then move on to the next exercise. Complete one circuit, recover for 90 seconds, then repeat the circuit three times.

■ Alternating Lateral Raise with Leg Raise

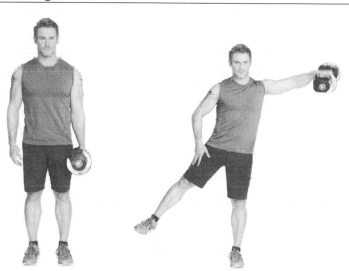

Setup: Stand with your feet shoulder-width apart, holding a dumbbell in each hand, palms facing in.

Action: Raise your left leg out to the side as you lift your right arm to the side until the dumbbell is at shoulder level. Lower the dumbbell as you return to start position. Repeat for 30 seconds, then switch sides.

■ Dumbbell Chest Fly with Glute Bridge

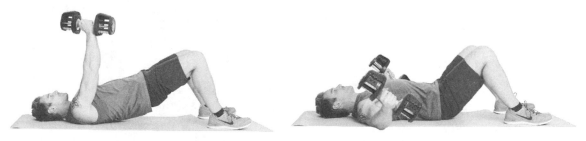

Setup: Lie back on an exercise bench or mat with your knees bent and your feet flat on the floor. Hold a dumbbell in each hand, palms facing in. Extend the dumbbells over your chest.

Action: Raise your hips so your body forms a straight line from your shoulder to your knees. Lower your hips back to the mat as you lower the dumbbells so they are even with your chest.

■ Reverse Lunge with Overhead Press

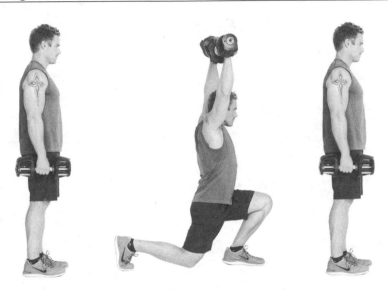

Setup: Stand with your feet shoulder-width apart, holding a dumbbell in each hand, arms hanging at your sides, palms facing each other.

Action: Curl the dumbbells up to your shoulders as you step your right foot back into a lunge. Press the dumbbells overhead, then press into your left heel to return to standing.

■ Quadruped Hip Extension

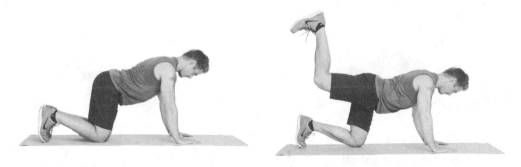

Setup: Place your hands under your shoulders and your knees under your hips.

Action: Lift your right leg behind you, keeping your knee bent at a 90-degree angle and pressing your right foot toward the ceiling. Return to start.

■ Reverse Crunch (see page 99 for photos)

Setup: Lie faceup on the floor. Place both hands by your hips, palms down.

Action: Keeping your knees and ankles together, bring your knees toward your chest. Squeeze your abdominals to lift your hips and legs toward the ceiling.

Lower your legs and repeat.

✱ *Jessie's Tip: Don't use your legs as momentum to lift up. Focus on the power coming from your abs.*

GETTING STARTED DAY 10: BUILD—STRENGTH TRAINING

■ Leg Day

Five sets of five reps
Recovery: 30–60 seconds between sets

■ Squat (Perfect Form Move, see page 57 for photos)

Setup: Stand with your feet hip-width apart, arms at your sides.

Action: Bend your knees like you're sitting in a chair until your thighs are nearly parallel to the floor. Slowly return to start position.

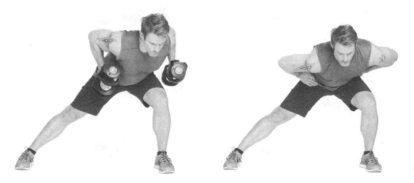

■ Lateral Lunge

Setup: Stand with your feet together, hands on hips.

Action: Take a big step to the right, keeping your left toes pointing straight ahead and bending your right knee until your thigh is almost parallel to the floor. Keep your left knee straight but not locked. Press off your right foot to return to start position. Complete all reps before switching sides.

▪ Dead Lift (see page 57 for photos)

Setup: Start with your feet shoulder-width apart, toes pointing straight ahead, arms down at your sides, and palms facing your thighs.

Action: Keeping your back slightly arched, hinge forward at your hips and lower your torso until it's almost parallel to the floor. Contract your hamstrings and glutes and push your hips forward to return to standing.

▪ Quadruped Hip Extension (see page 114 for photos)

Setup: Place your hands under your shoulders and your knees under your hips.

Action: Lift your right leg behind you, keeping your knee bent at a 90-degree angle and pressing your right foot toward the ceiling. Return to start. Repeat for 30 seconds, then switch sides.

▪ Glute Bridge

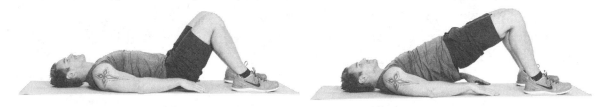

Setup: Lie on your back with your knees bent and your feet flat on the floor.

Action: Lift your hips off the floor, press your heels into the floor, and contract your glutes.

GETTING STARTED DAY 11: BURN—ATHLETIC TRAINING

▪ HIIT Athletic Training

Alternate 30 seconds of work and 30 seconds recovery.

■ Reverse Lunge with Rotation

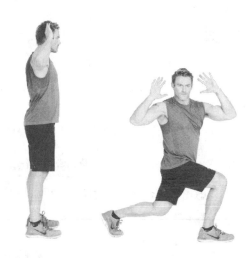

Setup: Stand with your feet shoulder-width apart with your fingertips by your ears.

Action: Take a step backward with your right leg, lowering your right knee toward the floor. Keeping your hips facing forward and chest open, twist to the left. Return to face forward, then push back to starting position. Continue, alternating legs.

■ Jump Rope (see page 90 for photos)

Setup: Stand with your feet together and imagine you are holding jump rope handles.

Action: Push off the floor with the balls of your feet, land softly, and push off again.

■ Speed Skate (see page 91 for photos)

Setup: Stand with your feet hip-width apart, knees slightly bent.

Action: Leap or step to the right side and land on your right leg, reaching down with your left hand toward your right knee or toes. Leap or step to the left side and land on your left leg, reaching down with your right hand toward your left knee or toes.

■ Jumping Jack (see page 102 for photos)

Setup: Start standing with your arms by your sides.

Action: Jump your legs out to the sides as you bring your arms overhead. Jump your feet back together and return arms to your sides.

■ Half Jack (see page 103 for photos)

Setup: Start standing with your arms by your sides.

Action: Tap your right leg out to your right side as you reach your left arm up to the ceiling. Repeat on the other side.

GETTING STARTED DAY 12: BUILD—STRENGTH TRAINING

■ Full Body

Five sets of five reps
Recovery: 30–60 seconds between sets

■ Squat with Knee Raise Balance

Setup: Stand with your feet hip-width apart, arms at your sides.

Action: Bend your knees like you're sitting in a chair until your thighs are nearly parallel to the floor. Keeping your weight on your left foot, raise your right knee toward your chest as you stand up. Return to squat position. Repeat five times on the right side, then five times on the left side.

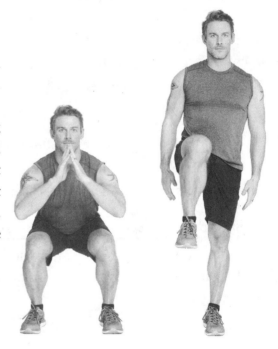

■ Knee Push-up (Perfect Form Move, see page 86 for photos)

Setup: Start on your hands and knees. Straighten your torso and place your hands directly underneath your shoulders, slightly wider than your shoulders, and rest on your knees.

Action: Bend your elbows and slowly lower your chest toward the floor. Push up to start position.

■ Reverse Lunge with Rotation (see page 117 for photos)

Setup: Stand with your feet shoulder-width apart with your fingertips by your ears.

Action: Take a step backward with your right leg, lowering your right knee toward the floor. Keeping your hips facing forward and chest open, twist to the left. Return to face forward, then push back to starting position.

■ **Dumbbell Chest Fly with Glute Bridge** (see page 113 for photos)

Setup: Lie back on an exercise bench or mat with your knees bent and your feet flat on the floor. Hold a dumbbell in each hand, palms facing in. Extend the dumbbells over your chest.

Action: Raise your hips so your body forms a straight line from your shoulders to your knees. Lower your hips back to the mat as you lower the dumbbells so they are even with your chest.

■ **Squat with Dumbbell Overhead Press** (see page 104 for photos)

Setup: Stand with your feet hip-width apart, holding a dumbbell in each hand at your shoulders, palms facing in.

Action: Bend your knees like you're sitting in a chair until your thighs are nearly parallel to the floor. As you rise out of the squat, lift the dumbbells overhead until they are about an inch apart. Lower the dumbbells as you return to start position.

GETTING STARTED DAY 13: SLOW BURN AND FLOW

Walk briskly or jog for 20 minutes today. This should be at a somewhat higher intensity than you were able to do during the first four Cleanse eating days. If you have a timer or step tracker on your phone or wristwatch, try using it and see if you can't cover 1½ miles in 20 minutes. One mile in about 15 minutes is very brisk. If you are able to, intersperse your brisk walking with a light jog when you can. Start by walking for a few minutes, then jog at a pace such that you could still have a conversation with someone. When you feel like you're working too hard to do that, or even if you're noticing that you're breathing heavily, slow down to a walk and keep walking until you feel completely recovered. You might alternate between walking and jogging four times each in 20 minutes, or even 10 times—anything is fine.

PART 2: FLOW

■ **Downward-Facing Dog** (see page 95 for photos)

Setup: Begin in plank. As you inhale, spread your fingers wide and press both palms firmly into the mat while simultaneously tucking your toes under. As you exhale, begin to draw your hips toward the ceiling, making the shape of an inverted V. Your head and neck should be between your upper arms. Bend your knees as much as you need to while maintaining equal weight on your hands and feet. Hold for three to five breath cycles.

Flow from Downward-Facing Dog into Low Lunge.

■ Low Lunge (see page 96 for photos)

Step your right foot between your hands, coming into a low lunge position. Shift your weight forward slightly to allow your right thigh to become parallel to the floor while remaining on the ball of your back foot (that should be your left foot).

Flow from Low Lunge into Warrior I.

■ Warrior I (see page 96 for photos)

Keeping your front foot facing forward, turn your back foot slightly outward and let your back foot rest flat at a 45-degree angle. Reach your arms overhead so they are parallel to one another. Your hips should still be facing forward as you lower your shoulders away from your ears and lift your core as you bend your front knee (your right knee) into a 90-degree angle. Hold this position for three to five breath cycles.

Flow from Warrior I into Warrior II.

■ Warrior II (see page 97 for photos)

Rotate your weight to the left and bring your arms straight out to your sides, parallel to the floor. Although the position of your feet does not change, your hips should now face the left. Your front leg (your right leg) should be bent while your back (left leg) is straight. This is Warrior II pose. Hold it for three to five breath cycles.

Flow from Warrior II into Side Angle.

■ Side Angle (see page 97 for photos)

Drop your right forearm on your right thigh and tilt your torso open, so that your left hand is now up in the air, reaching for the ceiling. Hold for three to five breath cycles.

Repeat this sequence on the other side. This means that you'll step back with your right leg back into Downward-Facing Dog and repeat the entire flow on your left side.

Continue to alternate sets between sides two to five times.

GETTING STARTED DAY 14: BUILD—STRENGTH TRAINING

■ Push Day

Five sets of five reps
Recovery: 30–60 seconds between sets

■ Knee Push-up (see page 86 for photos)

Setup: Start on your hands and knees. Straighten your torso and place your hands directly underneath your shoulders, slightly wider than your shoulders, and rest on your knees.

Action: Bend your elbows and slowly lower your chest toward the floor. Push up to start position.

■ Shoulder Press (see page 107 for photos)

Setup: Stand with your feet shoulder-width apart, holding a dumbbell in each hand at shoulder level.

Action: Press the dumbbells overhead, keeping your arms in line with your ears. Slowly lower your arms to shoulder height.

■ Triceps Dip (see page 87 for photos)

Setup: Sit on the edge of bench or sturdy chair, hands grasping the seat on either side of your hips. Keep your feet flat on the floor with your knees bent and bring your hips off the edge of the bench or chair.

Action: Bend your elbows and lower your hips toward the floor. Straighten your arms and return to starting position.

■ Lateral Raise (see page 108 for photos)

Setup: Stand with your feet shoulder-width apart, holding a dumbbell in each hand with palms facing in.

Action: Keeping your arms straight but not locked, raise the dumbbells out to the side in line with your shoulders. Lower the dumbbells to starting position.

∎ Dumbbell Chest Fly (see page 108 for photos)

Setup: Lie back on an exercise bench or mat with a dumbbell in each hand, palms facing in. Extend the dumbbells over your chest.

Action: Lower your arms until the weights are even with your chest. Press the dumbbells back to starting position.

GETTING STARTED DAY 15: BURN—ATHLETIC TRAINING

∎ HIIT Athletic Training

Alternate 30 seconds of work and 30 seconds of recovery.

Do all four exercises 30 seconds on, then 30 seconds off, one after the other, then recover for 1 minute. Repeat the circuit four times.

∎ Pass the Ball, Shoot the Ball (see page 90 for photos)

Setup: Stand with your feet slightly wider than hip-width apart, knees slightly bent and hands at chest level.

Action: Imagine you are holding a basketball at your chest. Pivot to your right side and push your arms out as if passing the ball. Come back to starting position and jump up or lift up on your toes and pretend to shoot the ball. Repeat on the other side.

∎ Side Shuffle (see page 122 for photos)

Setup: Stand with your feet shoulder-width apart, knees slightly bent.

Action: Take a large step out to your right with your right foot, bring your left foot over to meet the right, take another large step to the right with your right foot, then bend your knees to tap the floor with your left hand. Repeat in the other direction.

∎ Lunge Kick Lunge (see page 109 for photos)

Setup: Stand with feet shoulder-width apart with knees slightly bent.

Action: Step back with your right foot into a lunge, press off the ball of your right foot, and kick your right leg forward.

Repeat for 30 seconds, switching sides on the next circuit.

✴ *Jessie's Tip: Don't worry about how high you kick. Focus on your balance and keeping your core engaged.*

■ Alternating Elbow to Knee (see page 110 for photos)

Setup: Stand with your feet shoulder-width apart and extend your right arm up and your left leg to the side.

Action: Lower your right elbow and raise your left knee, crunching them together on a diagonal line. Repeat for 30 seconds, switching sides on the next circuit.

GETTING STARTED DAY 16: BUILD—STRENGTH TRAINING

■ Pull Day

Five sets of five reps
Recovery: 30–60 seconds between sets

■ Dumbbell Row (see page 110 for photos)

Setup: Stand with your feet hip-width apart with a dumbbell in each hand, palms facing in. Hinge forward to a 45-degree angle from the hips, keeping your back long and knees slightly bent.

Action: Pull the dumbbells up until your elbows pass your torso. Lower to starting position.

■ Biceps Curl (see page 111 for photos)

Setup: Stand with your feet hip-width apart, holding a dumbbell in each hand, palms facing forward.

Action: Curl the weights toward your shoulders, then return to the starting position.

■ Lat Pullover (see page 111 for photos)

Setup: Lie faceup on a bench or mat. Hold a dumbbell in each hand over your chest, keeping your elbows slightly bent.

Action: Extend your arms over your chest, palms facing in. Keeping your elbows slightly bent, lower the dumbbells in an arc back over your head toward the floor. Bring your elbows level with your head, then return to start position.

■ Resistance Band Row (see page 112 for photos)

Setup: Attach the resistance band door attachment at chest height. Stand facing the door, holding both handles and with your knees slightly bent.

Action: Reach forward with your arms in line with your shoulders. Pull the band back until your elbows pass your torso. Return to start.

■ Back Extension with Alternating Arm Raise (see page 112 for photos)

Setup: Lie facedown on a mat with your arms and legs extended.

Action: Keeping your neck in line with your spine, lift your right leg and left arm off the mat. Return to start, and repeat on the other side.

GETTING STARTED DAY 17: BURN—METABOLIC TRAINING

■ 5×5: Five Exercises, 1 Minute Each Exercise, Five Times

Perform each exercise for 60 seconds, then move on to the next exercise. Complete one circuit and recover for 90 seconds, then repeat the circuit five times.

■ Squat with Dumbbell Overhead Press (see page 104 for photos)

Setup: Stand with your feet hip-width apart, holding a dumbbell in each hand at your shoulders, palms facing in.

Action: Bend your knees like you're sitting in a chair until your thighs are nearly parallel to the floor. As you rise out of the squat, lift the dumbbells overhead until they are about an inch apart. Lower the dumbbells as you return to start position.

■ Alternating Step-up (see page 105 for photos)

Setup: Stand with your feet hip-width apart in front of a bench.

Action: Place your right foot on the bench so that your foot is completely on the bench. Push through your right heel to raise your body onto the bench, tap your left foot to the top of the bench, and return to starting position, then step up with your left foot. Continue, alternating legs.

■ Sumo Squat Biceps Curl (see page 105 for photos)

Setup: Stand with your feet slightly wider than hip-width apart, toes out, arms in front of you, holding a dumbbell in each hand, palms facing inward.

Action: Bend your knees and lower your body until your thighs are parallel to the floor. Push yourself back up as you rotate your wrists outward and curl the dumbbells to your shoulders.

■ Reverse Lunge Lateral Raise (see page 106 for photos)

Setup: Stand with your feet shoulder-width apart with a dumbbell in each hand, arms down at your sides, palms facing each other.

Action: Take a step backward with your right leg, lowering your right knee toward the floor and simultaneously lifting the dumbbells out to the sides to shoulder level. Return to starting position. Continue, alternating legs.

■ Crunch (see page 98 for photos)

Setup: Lie faceup with your knees bent, feet flat on the floor, and hands behind your head with fingertips lightly touching.

Action: Lift your shoulders off the floor until you feel a tight contraction on your abdominals. Return to starting position and repeat.

GETTING STARTED DAY 18: BUILD—STRENGTH TRAINING

■ Leg Day

Five sets of five reps
Recovery: 30–60 seconds between sets

■ Squat (see page 57 for photos)

Setup: Stand with your feet hip-width apart, arms at your sides.

Action: Bend your knees like you're sitting in a chair until your thighs are nearly parallel to the floor. Slowly return to start position

■ Lateral Lunge (see page 115 for photos)

Setup: Stand with your feet together, hands on hips.

Action: Take a big step to the right, keeping your left toes pointing straight ahead and bending your right knee until your thigh is almost parallel to the floor. Keep your left knee straight but not locked. Press off your right foot to return to start position. Complete all reps before switching sides.

■ Dead Lift (see page 57 for photos)

Setup: Start with your feet shoulder-width apart, toes pointing straight ahead, arms down at your sides, and palms facing your thighs.

Action: Keeping your back slightly arched, hinge forward at your hips and lower your torso until it's almost parallel to the floor. Contract your hamstrings and glutes and push your hips forward to return to standing.

■ Quadruped Hip Extension (see page 114 for photos)

Setup: Place your hands under your shoulders and your knees under your hips.

Action: Lift your right leg behind you, keeping your knee bent at a 90-degree angle and pressing your right foot toward the ceiling. Return to start. Repeat for 30 seconds, then switch sides.

■ Glute Bridge (see page 116 for photos)

Setup: Lie on your back with your knees bent and your feet flat on the floor.

Action: Lift your hips off the floor, press your heels into the floor, and contract your glutes.

GETTING STARTED DAY 19: BURN—ATHLETIC TRAINING

■ HIIT Athletic Training

Alternate 30 seconds of work and 30 seconds of recovery.

■ Reverse Lunge with Rotation (see page 117 for photos)

Setup: Stand with your feet shoulder-width apart with your fingertips by your ears.

Action: Take a step backward with your right leg, lowering your right knee toward the floor. Keeping your hips facing forward and chest open, twist to the left. Return to face forward, then push back to starting position. Continue, alternating legs.

■ Jump Rope (see page 90 for photos)

Setup: Stand with your feet together, and imagine you are holding jump rope handles.

Action: Push off the floor with the balls of your feet, land softly, and push off again.

■ Speed Skate (see page 91 for photos)

Setup: Stand with your feet hip-width apart, knees slightly bent.

Action: Leap or step to the right side and land on your right leg, reaching down with your left hand toward your right knee or toes. Leap or step to the left side and land on your left leg, reaching down with your right hand toward your left knee or toes.

▪ Jumping Jack (see page 102 for photos)

Setup: Start standing with your arms by your sides.

Action: Jump your legs out to the sides as you bring your arms overhead. Jump your feet back together and return arms to your sides.

▪ Half Jacks (see page 103 for photos)

Setup: Start standing with your arms by your sides.

Action: Tap your right leg out to your right side as you reach your left arm up to the ceiling. Repeat on the other side.

GETTING STARTED DAY 20: BUILD—STRENGTH TRAINING

▪ Full Body

Five sets of five reps
Recovery: 30–60 seconds between sets

▪ Squat with Knee Raise Balance (see page 118 for photos)

Setup: Stand with your feet hip-width apart, arms at your sides.

Action: Bend your knees like you're sitting in a chair until your thighs are nearly parallel to the floor. Keeping your weight on your left foot, raise your right knee toward your chest as you stand up. Return to squat position. Repeat five times on the right side, then five times on the left side.

▪ Knee Push-up (see page 86 for photos)

Setup: Start on your hands and knees. Straighten your torso and place your hands directly underneath your shoulders, slightly wider than your shoulders, and rest on your knees.

Action: Bend your elbows and slowly lower your chest toward the floor. Push up to start position.

▪ Reverse Lunge with Rotation (see page 117 for photos)

Setup: Stand with your feet shoulder-width apart with your fingertips by your ears.

Action: Take a step backward with your right leg, lowering your right knee toward the floor. Keeping your hips facing forward and chest open, twist to the left. Return to face forward, then push back to starting position.

■ Dumbbell Chest Fly with Glute Bridge (see page 113 for photos)

Setup: Lie back on an exercise bench or mat with your knees bent and your feet flat on the floor. Hold a dumbbell in each hand, palms facing in. Extend the dumbbells over your chest.

Action: Raise your hips so your body forms a straight line from your shoulders to your knees. Lower your hips back to the mat as you lower the dumbbells so they are even with your chest.

■ Squat with Dumbbell Overhead Press (see page 104 for photos)

Setup: Stand with your feet hip-width apart, holding a dumbbell in each hand at your shoulders, palms facing in.

Action: Bend your knees like you're sitting in a chair until your thighs are nearly parallel to the floor. As you rise out of the squat, lift the dumbbells overhead until they are about an inch apart. Lower the dumbbells as you return to start position.

GETTING STARTED DAY 21: BURN—METABOLIC TRAINING

Perform each exercise for 60 seconds, then move on to the next exercise. Complete one circuit and recover for 90 seconds, then repeat the circuit three times.

■ Alternating Lateral Raise with Leg Raise (see page 113 for photos)

Setup: Stand with your feet shoulder-width apart, holding a dumbbell in each hand, palms facing in.

Action: Raise your left leg out to the side as you lift your right arm to the side until the dumbbell is at shoulder level. Lower the dumbbell as you return to start position. Repeat for 30 seconds, then switch sides.

■ Dumbbell Chest Fly with Glute Bridge (see page 113 for photos)

Setup: Lie back on an exercise bench or mat with your knees bent and your feet flat on the floor. Hold a dumbbell in each hand, palms facing in. Extend the dumbbells over your chest.

Action: Raise your hips so your body forms a straight line from your shoulder to your knees. Lower hips back to the mat as you lower the dumbbells so they are even with your chest.

■ Reverse Lunge with Overhead Press (see page 114 for photos)

Setup: Stand with your feet shoulder-width apart, holding a dumbbell in each hand, arms hanging at your sides, palms facing each other.

Action: Curl the dumbbells up to your shoulders as you step your right foot back into a lunge. Press the dumbbells overhead, then press into your left heel to return to standing.

■ Quadruped Hip Extension (see page 114 for photos)

Setup: Place your hands under your shoulders and your knees under your hips.

Action: Lift your right leg behind you, keeping your knee bent at a 90-degree angle and pressing your right foot toward the ceiling. Return to start. Repeat for 30 seconds, then switch sides.

■ Reverse Crunch (see page 99 for photos)

Setup: Lie faceup on the floor. Place both hands by your hips, palms down.

Action: Keeping your knees and ankles together, bring your knees toward your chest. Squeeze your abdominals to lift your hips and legs toward the ceiling.

Lower your legs and repeat.

✱ *Jessie's Tip: Don't use your legs as momentum to lift up. Focus on the power coming from your abs.*

RAMP IT UP (INTERMEDIATE)

Wake-up Workout

This 4-minute circuit will get you ready and energized for a healthy day. You will be doing each exercise for 20 seconds, recovering for 10 seconds, then moving on to the next exercise. Repeat the circuit two times.

■ **Jumping Jack (see page 102 for photos)**

Setup: Start standing with your arms by your sides.

Action: Jump your legs out to the sides as you bring your arms overhead. Jump your feet back together and return arms to your sides.

■ **Push-up (see page 58 for photos)**

Setup: Start on the floor lying on your stomach, with your hands close to your chest and your elbows at a 45-degree angle.

Action: Raise yourself off the floor until your arms are fully extended. Your hands and the balls of your feet should support your weight. Keep a straight line from your head to your heels, contracting your abdominals and glutes so your hips don't sag. Lower your chest to the floor. Repeat.

■ **Alternating Lateral Lunge (see page 94 for photos)**

Setup: Stand with your feet together, arms at your sides.

Action: Take a big step to the right, keeping your left toes pointing straight ahead and bending your right knee until your thigh is almost parallel to the floor. Keep your left knee straight but not locked. Press off your right foot to return to start position. Repeat on the other leg.

■ **Plank with Alternating Knee Cross**

Setup: Start in push-up position with hands directly under shoulders.

Action: Turn your right knee in and bring it toward your left shoulder. Return to start and repeat on other side.

RAMP IT UP DAY 5: BURN—METABOLIC TRAINING

■ Five Exercises, 1 Minute Each Exercise, Repeat Circuit Three Times

Perform each exercise for 60 seconds, then move on to the next exercise. Complete one circuit, recover for 90 seconds, then repeat the circuit three times.

■ Dumbbell Step-up with Biceps Curl

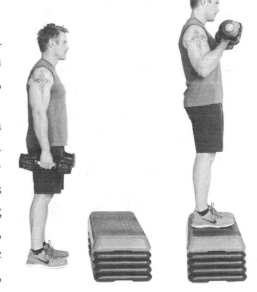

Setup: Stand with your feet hip-width apart in front of a bench. Hold a dumbbell in each hand, arms hanging by your side, palms facing in.

Action: Place your right foot on the bench so that your foot is completely on the bench. Push through your right heel to raise your body onto the bench, as you lift up curl dumbbells up toward your shoulders with palms facing in, tap your left foot to the top of the bench, and return to starting position as you lower the dumbbells. Repeat on right side for 30 seconds, then change legs.

■ Dumbbell Wood Chop

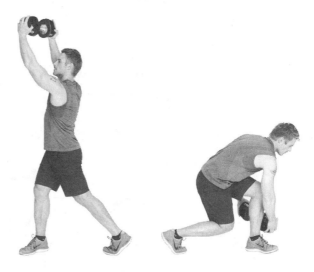

Setup: Stand with feet wider than hip-width apart, holding a dumbbell with both hands high above your right shoulder, arms straight with a slight bend at your elbows. Rotate your torso to the right.

Action: Swing the dumbbell down to the outside of your left knee as you rotate to the left, pivoting on your right toes and bending both knees. Return to start, repeat for 30 seconds, then switch sides.

■ Resistance Band Chest Fly

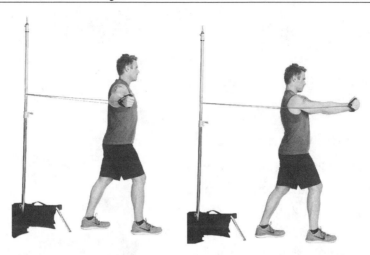

Setup: Attach the resistance band door attachment at chest height. Stand with your back facing the door, one handle in each hand. Extend your arms out with your palms facing each other. Step your right foot forward into a lunge until the band is taut.

Action: Pull your hands together, maintaining a slight bend in your elbows. Return to start and repeat for 30 seconds with the right leg forward. Switch legs and repeat for 30 seconds.

■ Squat with Dumbbell Overhead Press

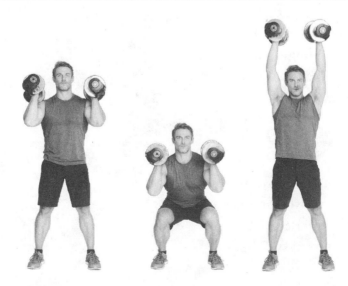

Setup: Stand with your feet hip-width apart, holding a dumbbell in each hand at your shoulders, palms facing in.

Action: Bend your knees like you're sitting in a chair until your thighs are nearly parallel to the floor. As you rise out of the squat, lift the dumbbells overhead until they are about an inch apart. Lower the dumbbells as you return to start position.

■ Russian Twist with Dumbbell

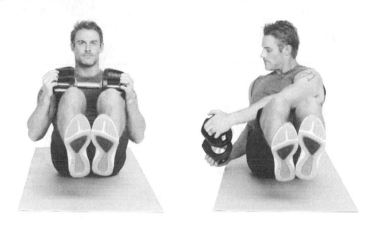

Setup: Sit on the floor with your knees bent and your heels about a foot from your hips. Hold a dumbbell with both hands in front of your chest. Lean back to a 45-degree angle without rounding your back.

Action: Holding the dumbbell at your chest with your elbows bent, pull your navel in toward your spine and rotate your torso to the right. Come back to center and rotate left.

RAMP IT UP DAY 6: BUILD—STRENGTH TRAINING

■ Push Day

Four sets of 10 reps
Recovery: 30–60 seconds between sets

■ Push-up (see page 58 for photos)

Setup: Start on the floor lying on your stomach, with your hands close to your chest and your elbows at a 45-degree angle.

Action: Raise yourself off the floor until your arms are fully extended. Your hands and the balls of your feet should support your weight. Keep a straight line from your head to your heels, contracting your abdominals and glutes so your hips don't sag. Lower your chest to the floor. Repeat.

▪ Triceps Extension

Setup: Stand with your feet shoulder-width apart, holding a dumbbell in each hand.

Action: Lift the dumbbells overhead and lower your hands behind your head, keeping elbows close to your ears. Push the dumbbells toward the ceiling without locking your elbows.

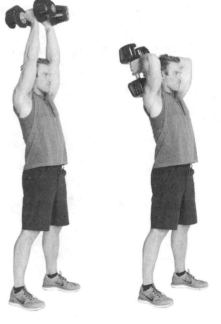

▪ Chest Press on Stability Ball

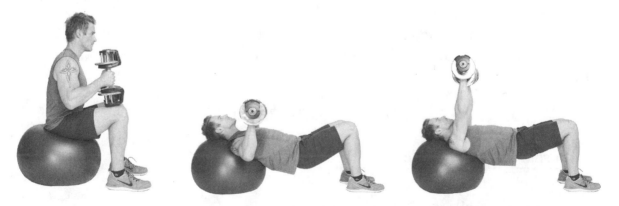

Setup: Sit on the stability ball, holding a dumbbell in each hand, with the dumbbells on your thighs. Slowly walk your feet forward and slide your torso down the ball until your head, shoulders, and upper back are on the ball. Your feet should be parallel and knees shoulder-width apart and bent at 90 degrees so your thighs and torso are parallel with the floor.

Action: Position the dumbbells over your chest with your palms facing forward. Press the dumbbells upward above your chest, elbows straight but not locked. Lower the dumbbells until they are level with your chest. Return to starting position.

▪ Triceps Extension on Stability Ball

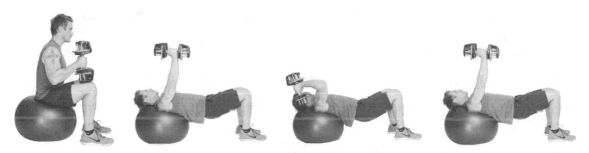

Setup: Sit on a stability ball with a dumbbell in each hand, your feet flat on the floor and the dumbbells resting on your thighs. Slowly walk your feet forward and slide your torso down the ball until your head, shoulders, and upper back are on the ball. Your feet should be parallel and knees shoulder-width apart and bent 90 degrees so your thighs and torso are parallel with the floor.

Action: Extend your arms at a 90-degree angle from the floor. Bend your elbows so your forearms are parallel to the floor. Straighten your arms without locking your elbows.

▪ Lateral Raise (see page 108 for photos)

Setup: Stand with your feet shoulder-width apart, holding a dumbbell in each hand, palms facing each other.

Action: Keeping your elbows slightly bent, raise the dumbbells to the sides until your arms are parallel with the floor. Lower to start position.

RAMP IT UP DAY 7: BURN—ATHLETIC TRAINING

▪ HIIT Athletic Training

Alternate 30 seconds of work with 30 seconds of recovery.

Do all four exercises 30 seconds on, then 30 seconds off, one after the other, then recover for 1 minute. Repeat the circuit four times.

■ High Knee Jog (see page 93 for photos)

Setup: Stand with your feet hip-width apart, knees slightly bent, arms at your sides.

Action: Bring your right knee up to hip level. Push off your left foot and switch legs, bringing your left leg up to hip level and landing on your right foot.

❋ *Jessie's Tip: Pump your arms like you are running, and always land with your knee slightly bent.*

■ Speed Skate (see page 91 for photos)

Setup: Stand with your feet hip-width apart, knees slightly bent.

Action: Leap to the right side and land on your right leg, reaching down with your left hand toward your right knee or toes. Leap to the left side and land on your left leg, reaching down with your right hand toward your left knee or toes.

■ Mountain Climber

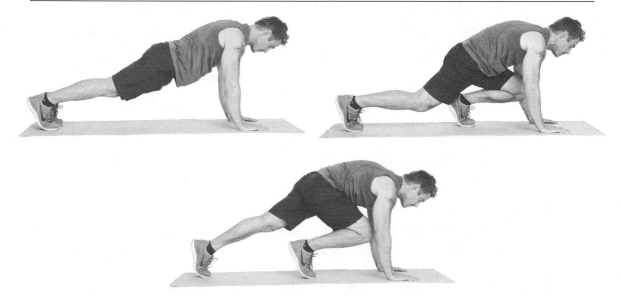

Setup: Assume a push-up position, arms extended, hands on the floor, legs extended.

Action: Keeping your body in a straight line, bring your right knee toward your chest. Return to start and repeat with your left leg.

■ Switch Jump Lunge

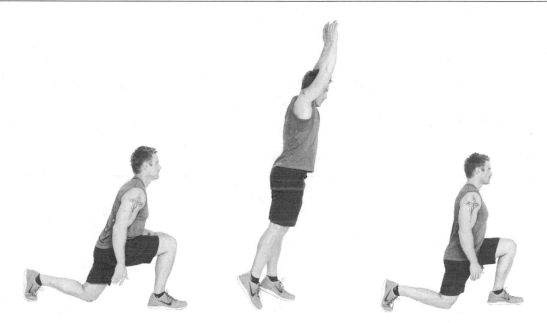

Setup: Lunge forward with your right thigh parallel to the floor, your left leg back.

Action: Jump up and switch leg positions. Land in a lunge with your left foot forward. Repeat on the other side.

RAMP IT UP DAY 8: BUILD—STRENGTH TRAINING

■ Pull Day

Four sets of 10 reps

Recovery: 30–60 seconds between sets

■ Bent-Over Row (see "Dumbbell Rows," page 110 for photos)

Setup: Stand with your feet hip-width apart, with a dumbbell in each hand, palms facing each other. Bend your knees slightly and bring your torso forward by bending at the waist, keeping your back straight and almost parallel to the floor.

Action: Lift the dumbbells to your sides until they pass your torso, keeping the dumbbells close to your body. Lower to start position.

■ Biceps Curl (see page 111 for photos)

Setup: Stand with your feet shoulder-width apart with a dumbbell in each hand, palms facing forward, arms hanging down at your sides.

Action: Keeping your elbows close to your torso, curl the dumbbells up toward your shoulders. Return to start position.

■ Resistance Band Lat Pull-down

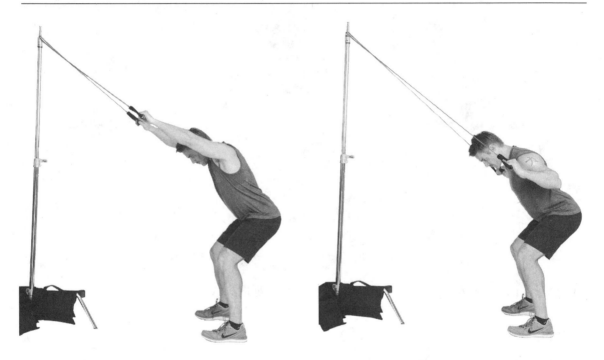

Setup: Attach the resistance band door attachment to the top of a door. Face the door and hold both handles. Back away from the door until your arms are straight.

Action: With your feet hip-width apart and knees slightly bent, lower your torso toward the floor and extend your arms past your head. Pull the handles toward you until they are taut. Bend your elbows out the sides until your hands are next to your shoulders. Return to start.

■ Resistance Band Biceps Curl

Setup: Stand with both feet on the resistance band, feet shoulder-width apart, holding a handle in each hand.

Action: Keeping your elbows close to your torso, curl the handles up toward your shoulders. Slowly lower the band and repeat.

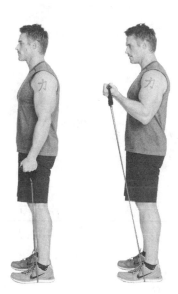

RAMP IT UP DAY 9: BURN—METABOLIC TRAINING

Perform each exercise for 60 seconds, then move on to the next exercise. Complete one circuit, recover for 90 seconds, then repeat the circuit three times.

■ Sumo Squat with Dumbbell: "Set It Down, Pick It Up"

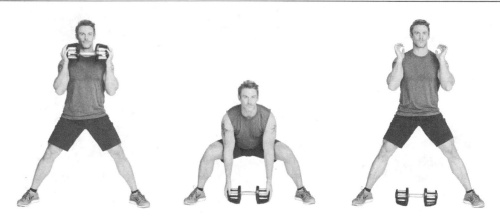

Setup: Stand with your feet slightly wider than hip-width apart, toes pointing out, holding a dumbbell with both hands at your chest.

Action: Bend your knees and lower your body until your thighs are parallel to the floor. Set the dumbbell on the floor and push yourself back up to standing. Squat down again and pick up the dumbbell.

■ Stability Ball Push-up

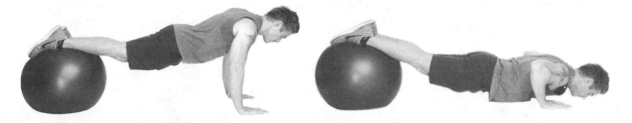

Setup: Come into a plank position, with your toes or shins resting on the ball. Place your hands shoulder-width apart.

Action: Bend your elbows to a 90-degree angle then press back to starting position.

■ Bench Jump Up and Over

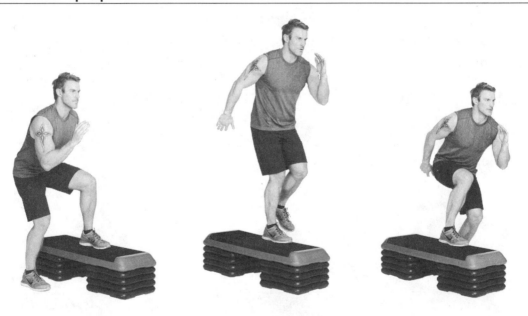

Setup: Stand to the left side of your bench with your left foot on the bench and your right foot on the floor.

Action: Bend both knees and push off your right foot, jumping over to the left and landing with your right foot on the bench. Repeat on the other side. Continue, alternating legs.

■ Lunge with Single Arm Row

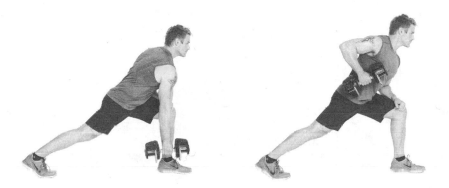

Setup: Hold a dumbbell in your right hand, step your left leg forward, and bend your left knee to 90 degrees. Lower your torso toward your left knee and place your left forearm on your left thigh. Push the dumbbell toward the floor.

Action: Row the dumbbell straight until your right elbow passes your torso. Return to starting position. Repeat for 30 seconds on the right side, then switch for 30 seconds on your left side.

■ Opposite Toe Touch Crunch

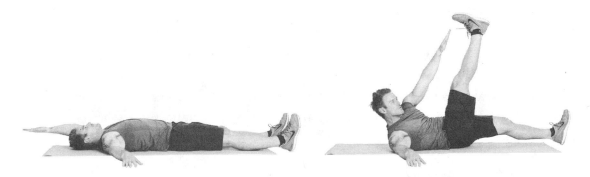

Setup: Lie on your back with your legs extended on the floor. Place your right hand on the floor.

Action: Lift your upper body off the floor as you reach your left arm up and across to your right toes. Return to starting position. Complete all reps on the right side, then switch sides.

RAMP IT UP DAY 10: BUILD—STRENGTH TRAINING

■ Leg Day

Four sets of 10 reps
Recovery: 30–60 seconds between sets

■ Dumbbell Goblet Squat

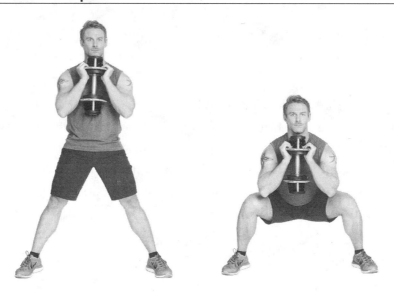

Setup: Stand with feet shoulder-width apart. Hold a dumbbell with both hands at chest level.

Action: Lower down into the bottom of a squat position. Keeping your heels pressing down into the floor, your back long, and your chest upright, push yourself back up to standing.

■ Dead Lift (see page 57 for photos)

Setup: Start with your feet shoulder-width apart, toes pointing straight ahead. Hold a pair of dumbbells in front of your thighs with your palms facing your body.

Action: Keeping your back straight, hinge forward at your hips and lower your torso until it's almost parallel to the floor, lowering the dumbbells toward your feet. Contract your hamstrings and glutes and push your hips forward to return to standing.

■ Dumbbell Step-up

Setup: Stand with your feet hip-width apart in front of a bench. Hold a dumbbell in each hand with your arms hanging down by your sides.

Action: Place your right foot on the bench so that your foot is completely on the bench. Push through your right heel to raise your body onto the bench, tap your left foot to the top of the bench, and return to starting position. Repeat 10 times on the right side, then on the left side.

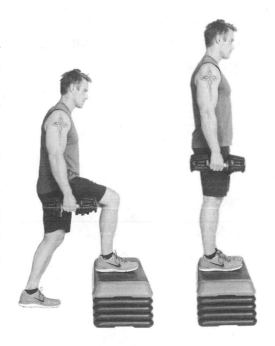

■ Split Squat off Bench (Bulgarian Squat)

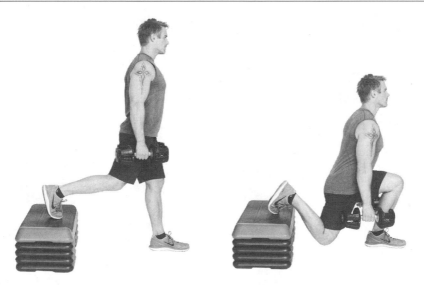

Setup: Stand about 3 feet in front of a bench, facing away from it. Hold a pair of dumbbells at your sides. Put your left foot on top of the bench and shift your weight to your right foot.

Action: Bend your right knee and lower your body toward the floor, keeping your right knee over the right ankle and bringing your right thigh parallel to the floor. Slowly stand back up to starting position.

▪ Glute Bridge on Bench

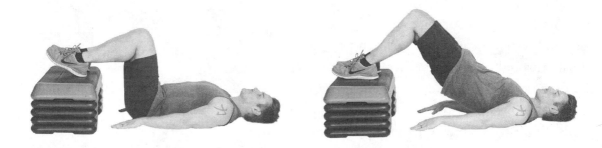

Setup: Lie on the floor with your feet on the bench, arms by your sides, and knees bent to 90 degrees.

Action: Press through your heels and lift your hips up, squeezing your glutes at the top. Slowly return to starting position.

RAMP IT UP DAY 11: BURN—ATHLETIC TRAINING

▪ HIIT Athletic Training

Alternate 30 seconds of work and 30 seconds of recovery.

▪ Jump Forward, Jog Back

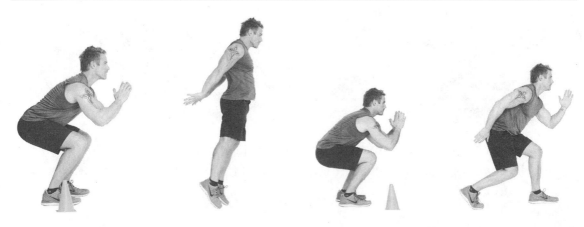

Setup: Start standing with your feet shoulder-width apart, knees slightly bent.

Action: Imagine there is a cone 3 feet in front of you. Squat down and jump forward toward the cone. Jog back to starting position.

■ Lunge Kick Lunge (see page 109 for photos)

Setup: Stand with feet shoulder-width apart with knees slightly bent.

Action: Step back with your right foot into a lunge, press off the ball of your right foot, and kick your right leg forward.

Repeat for 30 seconds, switching sides on the next circuit.

✳ *Jessie's Tip: Don't worry about how high you kick. Focus on your balance and keeping your core engaged.*

■ Plank Jack

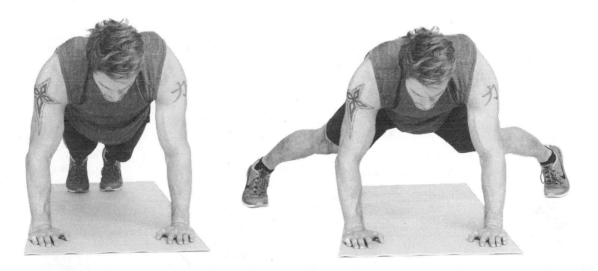

Setup: Assume a push-up position, arms extended, hands on the floor, legs extended with feet together.

Action: Jump your feet out to the sides, then back together.

■ Squat Jump

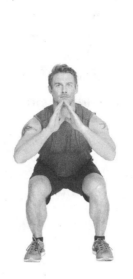
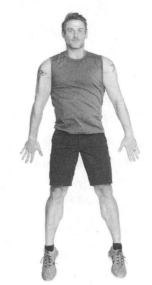

Setup: Stand with your feet shoulder-width apart, arms at your sides. Sit back into a squat until your thighs are parallel to the floor.

Action: Jump up explosively. Land with bent knees.

RAMP IT UP DAY 12: BUILD—STRENGTH TRAINING

■ Full Body

Four sets of 10 reps
Recovery: 30–60 seconds between sets

■ Side Step-up Shoulder Press Front Kick

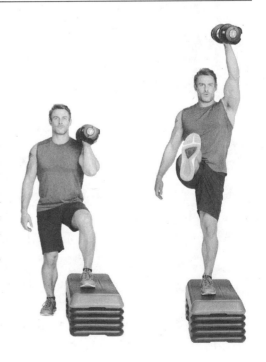

Setup: Stand with your right side next to a bench, holding a dumbbell in your right hand, elbow bent and palm facing in. Place your right foot on the step, bend your right knee, and extend your left arm out to the side.

Action: Straighten your right knee as you lift your left leg in front of you. Return to starting position. Complete all reps on the right side, then switch sides.

■ Plank to Side Plank

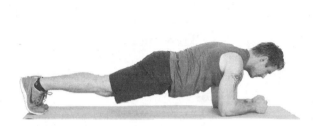
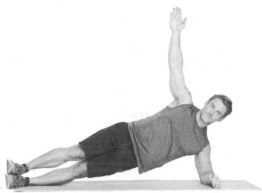

Setup: Get into a forearm plank.

Action: Keeping your body straight, transfer your weight to your left forearm and rotate your right arm toward the ceiling. Hold side plank for one breath. Return to forearm plank. (Ten reps is five planks on the right side and five planks on the left side.)

■ Lunge with Single Arm Row (see page 141 for photos)

Setup: Hold a dumbbell in your right hand, step your left leg forward, and bend your left knee to 90 degrees. Lower your torso toward your left knee and place your left forearm on your left thigh. Push the dumbbell toward the floor.

Action: Pull the dumbbell up until your right elbow passes your torso. Return to starting position. Repeat for 30 seconds on the right side, then switch for 30 seconds on your left side.

■ Forward Lunge with Biceps Curl

Setup: Stand with your feet hip-width apart, holding a dumbbell in each hand, arms down at your side, palms facing in.

Action: Take a step forward with your right foot and bend your right knee to 90 degrees, simultaneously curling the dumbbells up toward your shoulders. Push off your right foot and return to starting position. Complete all reps on the right side, then switch sides.

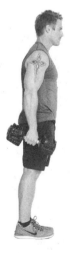
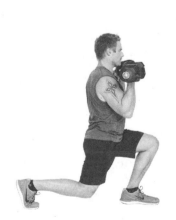

■ Opposite Toe Touch Crunch (see page 141 for photos)

Setup: Lie on your back with your legs extended on the floor. Place your right hand on the floor.

Action: Lift your upper body off the floor as you reach your left arm up and across to your right toes. Return to starting position. Complete all reps on the right side, then switch sides.

RAMP IT UP DAY 13: SLOW BURN AND FLOW

You should be alternating walking with jogging at a very comfortable pace for 30 minutes. Start by walking for a few minutes, then jog at a pace such that you could still have a conversation with someone. When you feel like you're working too hard to do that, or even if you're noticing that you're breathing heavily, slow down to a walk and keep walking until you feel completely recovered. You might alternate between walking and jogging four times each in 30 minutes, or even 10 times—anything is fine.

If you can, jog continuously for 30 minutes. You are not sprinting, so don't worry about your pace at all. You just want a comfortable, easy jog on relatively flat terrain. If you feel breathless after 10 or 15 minutes, slow down to a brisk walk until you are completely recovered.

PART 2: FLOW

■ Downward-Facing Dog (see page 95 for photos)

Setup: Begin on your hands and knees in plank position. As you inhale, spread your fingers wide and press both palms firmly into the mat while simultaneously tucking your toes under. As you exhale, begin to draw your hips toward the ceiling, making the shape of an inverted V. Your head and neck should be between your upper arms. Bend your knees as much as you need to while maintaining equal weight on your hands and feet. Hold for three to five breath cycles.

Flow from Downward-Facing Dog into Low Lunge.

■ Low Lunge (see page 96 for photos)

Step your right foot between your hands, coming into a low lunge position. Shift your weight forward slightly to allow your right thigh to become parallel to the floor while remaining on the ball of your back foot (that should be your left foot).

Flow from Low Lunge into Warrior I.

■ Warrior I (see page 96 for photos)

Keeping your front foot facing forward, turn your back foot slightly outward and let your back foot rest flat at a 45-degree angle. Reach your arms overhead so they are parallel to one another. Your hips should still be facing forward as you lower your shoulders away from your ears and lift your core as you bend your front knee (your right knee) into a 90-degree angle. Hold this position for three to five breath cycles.

Flow from Warrior I into Warrior II.

■ Warrior II (see page 97 for photos)

Rotate your weight to the left and bring your arms straight out to your sides, parallel to the floor. Although the position of your feet does not change, your hips should now face the left. Your front leg (your right leg) should be bent while your back (left leg) is straight. This is Warrior II pose. Hold it for three to five breath cycles.

Flow from Warrior II into Side Angle.

■ Side Angle (see page 97 for photos)

Drop your right forearm on your right thigh and tilt your torso open, so that your left hand is now up in the air, reaching for the ceiling. Hold for three to five breath cycles.

Repeat this sequence on the other side. This means that you'll step back with your right leg back into Downward-Facing Dog and repeat the entire flow on your left side.

Continue to alternate sets between sides two to five times.

RAMP IT UP DAY 14: BUILD—STRENGTH TRAINING

■ Push Day

Four sets of 10 reps
Recovery: 30–60 seconds between sets

■ Push-up (see page 58 for photos)

Setup: Start on the floor lying on your stomach, with your hands close to your chest and your elbows at a 45-degree angle.

Action: Raise yourself off the floor until your arms are fully extended. Your hands and the balls of your feet should support your weight. Keep a straight line from your head to your heels, contracting your abdominals and glutes so your hips don't sag. Lower your chest to the floor. Repeat.

■ Triceps Extension (see page 134 for photos)

Setup: Stand with your feet shoulder-width apart, holding a dumbbell in each hand.

Action: Lift the dumbbells overhead and lower your hands behind your head, keeping your elbows close to your ears. Push the dumbbells toward the ceiling without locking your elbows.

■ Chest Press on Stability Ball (see page 134 for photos)

Setup: Sit on the stability ball, holding a dumbbell in each hand, with the dumbbells on your thighs. Slowly walk your feet forward and slide your torso down the ball until your head, shoulders, and upper back are on the ball. Your feet should be parallel and knees shoulder-width apart and bent at 90 degrees so your thighs and torso are parallel with the floor.

Action: Position the dumbbells over your chest with your palms facing forward. Press the dumbbells upward above your chest, elbows straight but not locked. Lower the dumbbells until they are level with your chest. Return to starting position.

■ Triceps Extension on Stability Ball (see page 135 for photos)

Setup: Sit on a stability ball with a dumbbell in each hand, your feet flat on the floor and the dumbbells resting on your thighs. Slowly walk your feet forward and slide your torso down the ball until your head, shoulders, and upper back are on the ball. Your feet should be parallel and your knees shoulder-width apart and bent 90 degrees so your thighs and torso are parallel with the floor.

Action: Extend your arms to a 90-degree angle from the floor. Bend your elbows so your forearms are parallel to the floor. Straighten your arms without locking your elbows.

■ **Lateral Raise** (see page 108 for photos)

Setup: Stand with your feet shoulder-width apart, holding a dumbbell in each hand, palms facing each other.

Action: Keeping your elbows slightly bent, raise the dumbbells to the sides until your arms are parallel with the floor. Lower to start position.

RAMP IT UP DAY 15: BURN—ATHLETIC TRAINING

■ **HIIT Athletic Training**

Alternate 30 seconds of work with 30 seconds of recovery.

Do all four exercises 30 seconds on, then 30 seconds off, one after the other, then recover for 1 minute. Repeat the circuit four times.

■ **High Knee Jog** (see page 93 for photos)

Setup: Stand with your feet hip-width apart, knees slightly bent, arms at your sides.

Action: Bring your right knee up to hip level. Push off your left foot and switch legs, bringing your left leg up to hip level and landing on your right foot.

✱ *Jessie's Tip: Pump your arms like you are running, and always land with knee slightly bent.*

■ **Speed Skate** (see page 91 for photos)

Setup: Stand with your feet hip-width apart, knees slightly bent.

Action: Leap to the right side and land on your right leg, reaching down with your left hand toward your right knee or toes. Leap to the left side and land on your left leg, reaching down with your right hand toward your left knee or toes.

■ **Mountain Climber** (see page 136 for photos)

Setup: Assume a push-up position, arms extended, hands on the floor, legs extended.

Action: Keeping your body in a straight line, bring your right knee toward your chest. Return to start and repeat with your left leg.

■ **Switch Jump Lunge** (see page 137 for photos)

Setup: Lunge forward with your right thigh parallel to the floor, your left leg back.

Action: Jump up and switch leg positions. Land in a lunge with your left foot forward. Repeat on the other side.

RAMP IT UP DAY 16: BUILD—STRENGTH TRAINING

▪ Pull Day

Four sets of 10 reps
Recovery: 30–60 seconds between sets

▪ Bent-Over Row (see "Dumbbell Row," page 110 for photos)

Setup: Stand with your feet hip-width apart, with a dumbbell in each hand, palms facing each other. Bend your knees slightly and bring your torso forward by bending at the waist, keeping your back straight and almost parallel to the floor.

Action: Lift the dumbbells to your sides until they pass your torso, keeping the dumbbells close to your body. Lower to start position.

▪ Biceps Curl (see page 111 for photos)

Setup: Stand with your feet shoulder-width apart with a dumbbell in each hand, palms facing forward, arms hanging down at your sides.

Action: Keeping your elbows close to your torso, curl the dumbbells up toward your shoulders. Return to start position.

▪ Resistance Band Lat Pull-down (see page 138 for photos)

Setup: Attach the resistance band door attachment to the top of a door. Face the door and hold both handles. Back away from the door until your arms are straight.

Action: With your feet hip-width apart and knees slightly bent, lower your torso toward the floor and extend your arms past your head. Pull the handles toward you until they are taut. Bend your elbows out the sides until your hands are next to your shoulders. Return to start.

▪ Resistance Band Biceps Curl (see page 139 for photos)

Setup: Stand with both feet on the resistance band, feet shoulder-width apart, holding a handle in each hand.

Action: Keeping your elbows close to your torso, curl the handles up toward your shoulders. Slowly lower the band and repeat.

RAMP IT UP DAY 17: BURN—METABOLIC TRAINING

▪ Five Exercises, 1 Minute Each Exercise, Repeat Circuit Three Times

Perform each exercise for 60 seconds, then move on to the next exercise. Complete one circuit and recover for 90 seconds, then repeat the circuit three times.

▪ Dumbbell Step-up with Biceps Curl (see page 131 for photos)

Setup: Stand with your feet hip-width apart in front of a bench. Hold a dumbbell in each hand, arms hanging by your side and palms facing in.

Action: Place your right foot on the bench so that your foot is completely on the bench. Push through your right heel to raise your body onto the bench, and as you lift up curl the dumbbells up toward your shoulders with palms facing in. Tap your left foot to the top of the bench and return to starting position as you lower the dumbbells. Repeat on the right side for 30 seconds, then change legs.

▪ Dumbbell Wood Chop (see page 131 for photos)

Setup: Stand with feet wider than hip-width apart, holding a dumbbell with both hands high above your right shoulder, arms straight with a slight bend at your elbows. Rotate your torso to the right.

Action: Swing the dumbbell down to the outside of your left knee as you rotate to the left pivoting on your right toes and bending both knees. Return to start, repeat for 30 seconds, then switch sides.

▪ Resistance Band Chest Fly (see page 132 for photos)

Setup: Attach the resistance band door attachment at chest height. Stand with your back facing the door, one handle in each hand. Extend your arms out with your palms facing each other. Step your right foot forward into a lunge until the band is taut.

Action: Pull your hands together maintaining a slight bend in your elbows. Return to start and repeat for 30 seconds with the right leg forward. Switch legs and repeat for 30 seconds.

■ Squat with Dumbbell Overhead Press (see page 132 for photos)

Setup: Stand with your feet hip-width apart, holding a dumbbell in each hand at your shoulders, palms facing in.

Action: Bend your knees like you're sitting in a chair until your thighs are nearly parallel to the floor. As you rise out of the squat, lift the dumbbells overhead until they are about an inch apart. Lower the dumbbells as you return to start position.

■ Russian Twist with Dumbbell (see page 133 for photos)

Setup: Sit on the floor with your knees bent and your heels about a foot from your hips. Hold a dumbbell with both hands in front of your chest. Lean back to a 45-degree angle without rounding your back.

Action: Holding the dumbbell at your chest with your elbows bent, pull your navel in toward your spine and rotate your torso to the right. Come back to center and rotate left.

RAMP IT UP DAY 18: BUILD—STRENGTH TRAINING

■ Leg Day

Four sets of 10 reps
Recovery: 30–60 seconds between sets

■ Dumbbell Goblet Squat (see page 142 for photos)

Setup: Stand with feet shoulder-width apart. Hold a dumbbell with both hands at chest level.

Action: Lower down into the bottom of a squat position. Keeping your heels pressing down into the floor, your back long, and your chest upright, push yourself back up to standing.

■ Dead Lift (see page 57 for photos)

Setup: Start with your feet shoulder-width apart, toes pointing straight ahead. Hold a pair of dumbbells in front of your thighs with your palms facing your body.

Action: Keeping your back straight, hinge forward at your hips and lower your torso until it's almost parallel to the floor, lowering the dumbbells toward your feet. Contract your hamstrings and glutes and push your hips forward to return to standing.

■ **Dumbbell Step-up** (see page 143 for photos)

Setup: Stand with your feet hip-width apart in front of a bench. Hold a dumbbell in each hand arms hanging down by your sides.

Action: Place your right foot on the bench so that your foot is completely on the bench. Push through your right heel to raise your body onto the bench, tap your left foot to the top of the bench, and return to starting position. Repeat 10 times on the right side, then on the left side.

■ **Split Squat off Bench (Bulgarian Squat)** (see page 155 for photos)

Setup: Stand about 3 feet in front of a bench, facing away from it. Hold a pair of dumbbells at your sides. Put your left foot on top of the bench and shift your weight to your right foot.

Action: Bend your right knee and lower your body toward the floor, keeping your right knee over the right ankle and bringing your right thigh parallel to the floor. Slowly stand back up to starting position.

■ **Glute Bridge on Bench** (see page 144 for photos)

Setup: Lie on the floor with your feet on the bench, arms by your sides, and knees bent to 90 degrees.

Action: Press through your heels and lift your hips up, squeezing your glutes at the top. Slowly return to starting position.

RAMP IT UP DAY 19: BURN—ATHLETIC TRAINING

■ **HIIT Athletic Training**

Alternate 30 seconds of and work 30 seconds of recovery.

■ **Jump Forward, Jog Back** (see page 144 for photos)

Setup: Start standing with your feet shoulder-width apart, knees slightly bent.
Action: Imagine there is a cone 3 feet in front of you. Squat down and jump forward toward the cone. Jog back to starting position.

■ **Lunge Kick Lunge** (see page 109 for photos)

Setup: Stand with feet shoulder-width apart with knees slightly bent.

Action: Step back with your right foot into a lunge, press off the ball of your right foot, and kick your right leg forward.

Repeat for 30 seconds, switching sides on the next circuit.

✳ *Jessie's Tip: Don't worry about how high you kick. Focus on your balance and keeping your core engaged.*

■ **Plank Jack** (see page 145 for photos)

Setup: Assume a push-up position, arms extended, hands on the floor, and legs extended with feet together.

Action: Jump your feet out to the sides, then back together.

■ **Squat Jump** (see page 146 for photos)

Setup: Stand with feet shoulder-width apart, arms at your sides. Sit back into a squat until your thighs are parallel.

Action: Jump up explosively. Land with bent knees.

RAMP IT UP DAY 20: BUILD—STRENGTH TRAINING

■ **Full Body**

Four sets of 10 reps
Recovery: 30–60 seconds between sets

■ **Side Step-up Shoulder Press Front Kick** (see page 146 for photos)

Setup: Stand with your right side next to a bench, holding a dumbbell in your right hand, elbow bent and palm facing in. Place your right foot on the step, bend your right knee, and extend your left arm out to the side.

Action: Straighten your right knee as you lift your left leg in front of you. Return to starting position. Complete all reps on the right side, then switch sides.

■ **Plank to Side Plank** (see page 147 for photos)

Setup: Get into a forearm plank.

Action: Keeping your body straight, transfer your weight to your left forearm and rotate your right arm toward the ceiling. Hold side plank for one breath. Return to forearm plank. (Ten reps is five planks on the right side and five planks on the left side.)

◼ Lunge with Single Arm Row (see page 141 for photos)

Setup: Hold a dumbbell in your right hand, step your left leg forward, and bend your left knee to 90 degrees. Lower your torso toward your left knee and place your left forearm on your left thigh. Push the dumbbell toward the floor.

Action: Pull the dumbbell up until your right elbow passes your torso. Return to starting position. Repeat for 30 seconds on the right side, then switch for 30 seconds on your left side.

◼ Forward Lunge with Biceps Curl (see page 147 for photos)

Setup: Stand with your feet hip-width apart, holding a dumbbell in each hand, arms down at your side, palms facing in.

Action: Take a step forward with your right foot and bend your right knee to 90 degrees, simultaneously curling the dumbbells up toward your shoulders. Push off your right foot and return to starting position. Complete all reps on the right side, then switch sides.

◼ Opposite Toe Touch Crunch (see page 141 for photos)

Setup: Lie on your back with your legs extended on the floor. Place your right hand on the floor.

Action: Lift your upper body off the floor as you reach your left arm up and across to your right toes. Return to starting position. Complete all reps on the right side, then switch sides.

RAMP IT UP DAY 21: BURN—METABOLIC TRAINING

◼ Five Exercises, 1 Minute Each Exercise, Repeat Circuit Three Times

Perform each exercise for 60 seconds, then move on to the next exercise. Complete one circuit, recover for 90 seconds, then repeat the circuit three times.

■ Sumo Squat with Dumbbell: "Set It Down, Pick It Up"
(see page 139 for photos)

Setup: Stand with your feet slightly wider than hip-width apart, toes pointing out, holding a dumbbell with both hands at your chest.

Action: Bend your knees and lower your body until your thighs are parallel to the floor. Set the dumbbell on the floor and push yourself back up to standing. Squat down again and pick up the dumbbell.

■ Stability Ball Push-up (see page 140 for photos)

Setup: Come into a plank position, with your toes or shins resting on the ball. Place your hands shoulder-width apart.

Action: Bend your elbows to a 90-degree angle, then press back to starting position.

■ Bench Jump Up and Over (see page 140 for photos)

Setup: Stand to the left side of your bench with your left foot on the bench and your right foot on the floor.

Action: Bend both knees and push off your right foot, jumping over to the left and landing with your right foot on the bench. Repeat on the other side. Continue, alternating legs.

■ Lunge with Single Arm Row (see page 141 for photos)

Setup: Hold a dumbbell in your right hand, step your left leg forward and bend your left knee to 90 degrees. Lower your torso toward your left knee and place your left forearm on your left thigh. Push the dumbbell toward the floor.

Action: Row the dumbbell straight until your right elbow passes your torso. Return to starting position. Repeat for 30 seconds on the right side, then switch for 30 seconds on your left side.

■ Opposite Toe Touch Crunch (see page 141 for photos)

Setup: Lie on your back with your legs extended on the floor. Place your right hand on the floor.

Action: Lift your upper body off the floor as you reach your left arm up and across to your right toes. Return to starting position. Complete all reps on the right side, then switch sides.

FULL THROTTLE (ADVANCED)

Wake-up Workout

This 4-minute circuit will get you ready and energized for a healthy day. You will be doing each exercise for 20 seconds, recovering for 10 seconds, then moving on to the next exercise. Repeat the circuit two times.

■ **Jumping Jack (see page 102 for photos)**

Setup: Start standing with your arms by your sides.

Action: Jump your legs out to the sides as your bring your arms overhead.

Jump your feet back together and return arms to your sides.

■ **Squat Thrust (see page 93 for photos)**

Setup: Stand with your feet together, arms at your sides.

Action: Bend your knees and place your palms on the floor with your arms on the outside of your knees. Shift your weight onto your palms. Jump both feet back and land in plank position. Jump both feet forward and return to standing.

■ **Push-up (see page 58 for photos)**

Setup: Start on the floor lying on your stomach, with your hands close to your chest and your elbows at a 45-degree angle.

Action: Raise yourself off the floor until your arms are fully extended. Your hands and the balls of your feet should support your weight. Keep a straight line from your head to your heels, contracting your abdominals and glutes so your hips don't sag. Lower your chest to the floor. Repeat.

■ **Switch Jump Lunge (see page 137 for photos)**

Setup: Lunge forward with your right thigh parallel to the floor, your left leg back.

Action: Jump up and switch leg positions. Land in a lunge with your left foot forward. Repeat on the other side.

FULL THROTTLE DAY 5: BURN—METABOLIC TRAINING

∎ Five Exercises, 1 Minute Each Exercise, Repeat Circuit Three Times

Perform each exercise for 60 seconds, then move on to the next exercise. Complete one circuit, recover for 90 seconds, then repeat the circuit three times.

∎ Renegade Row

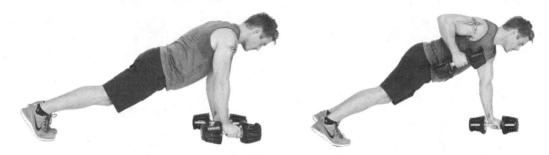

Setup: Assume the push-up position with your arms straight, feet slightly wider than shoulder-width, and hands holding a pair of dumbbells directly under your shoulders.

Action: Lift your left elbow toward the ceiling until your elbow passes your torso. Lower the weight, and repeat on the other side. Each row is counted as one rep.

∎ Squat Jump (see page 146 for photos)

Setup: Stand with your feet shoulder-width apart, arms at your sides. Sit back into a squat until your thighs are parallel to the floor.

Action: Jump up explosively. Land with bent knees.

∎ Stability Ball Push-up and Pike (see pages 140 and 100 for photos)

Setup: Start with your torso on the ball and hands and feet on the floor. Walk your hands forward until your legs are straight and your toes are on top of the ball. Hands are under shoulders.

Action: Lower yourself until your chest almost touches the floor. Press your upper body back to starting position. Keeping your legs straight, pull your feet toward your chest and push your hips toward the ceiling as the ball rolls in. Continue until your hips are directly under your shoulders. Slowly lower back to starting position. Continue alternating one push-up and one pike.

▪ Jump Forward, Jog Back (see page 144 for photos)

Setup: Start standing with your feet shoulder-width apart, knees slightly bent.

Action: Imagine there is a cone 3 feet in front of you. Squat down and jump forward toward the cone. Jog back to starting position.

▪ V Sit with Incline Dumbbell Chest Press

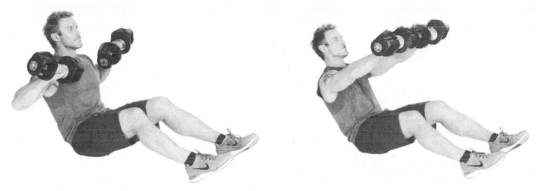

Setup: Sit on the floor with your feet flat, holding a light dumbbell in each hand in front of your shoulders. Lean back so your torso is at a 45-degree angle.

Action: Engage your core and press the dumbbells away from your body until your arms are straight. Return to start.

FULL THROTTLE DAY 6: BUILD—STRENGTH TRAINING

▪ Push Day

Four sets of 15 reps
Recovery: 30–60 seconds between sets

▪ Stability Ball Push-up (see page 140 for photos)

Setup: Come into a plank position, with your toes or shins resting on the ball. Place your hands shoulder-width apart.

Action: Bend your elbows to a 90-degree angle, then press back to starting position.

■ Pistol Squat

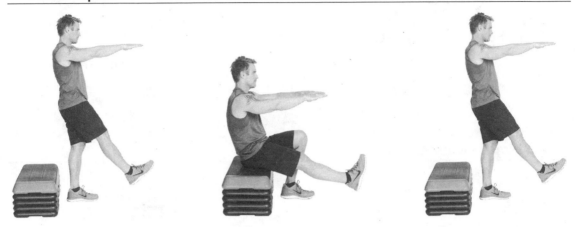

Setup: Stand on your right foot with your left leg extended in front of you.

Action: Bend your right knee and squat down as far as you can while keeping your left leg lifted. Extend your right leg to return to start position.

■ Chest Press on Bench

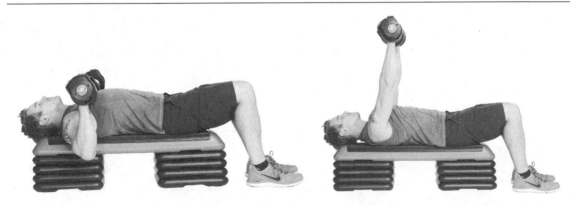

Setup: Lie on a bench with a dumbbell in each hand and your feet flat on the floor. Position dumbbells over your chest with your palms facing forward.

Action: Press the dumbbells upward above your chest, elbows straight but not locked. Lower the dumbbells until they are level with your chest. Return to starting position.

■ Lying Triceps Extensions on the Bench

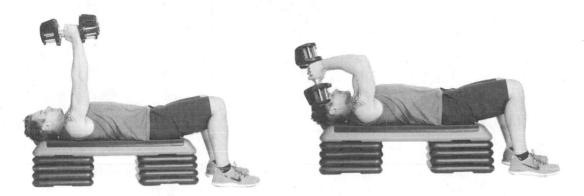

Setup: Lie on a bench, holding a dumbbell in each hand. Extend your arms to a 90-degree angle from the floor.

Action: Bend your elbows so your forearms are parallel to the floor. Straighten your arms without locking your elbows.

■ Front Raise/Lateral Raise

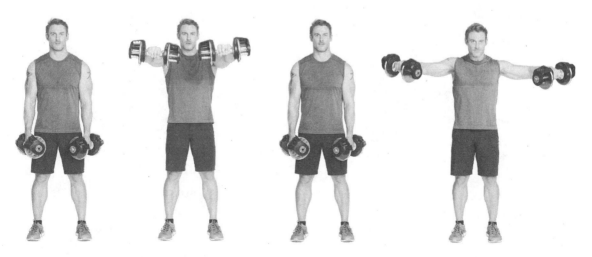

Setup: Stand with feet shoulder-width apart, holding a dumbbell in each hand, palms facing each other.

Action: Keeping your elbows slightly bent, raise the dumbbells to the sides until your arms are parallel with the floor. Lower to start position. Turn your hands so your palms face your thighs, and raise the dumbbells forward until they are parallel to the floor. One front and one lateral raise are counted as one repetition.

FULL THROTTLE DAY 7: BURN—ATHLETIC TRAINING

■ Tabata Training

20 seconds work, 10 seconds recovery
Repeat one exercise four times for 20 seconds on and 10 seconds of rest.
Recover 30–60 seconds before moving on to the next exercise.

■ Speed Skate (see page 91 for photos)

Setup: Stand with your feet hip-width apart, knees slightly bent.
Action: Leap to the right side and land on your right leg, reaching down with your left hand toward your right knee or toes. Leap to the left side and land on your left leg, reaching down with your right hand toward your left knee or toes.

■ Spiderman Push-up

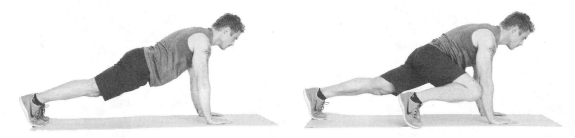

Setup: Start in a plank position with your hands under your shoulders.
Action: Bring your right knee outward toward your right elbow. Return to start position, and repeat with left leg.

■ 180-Degree Jump

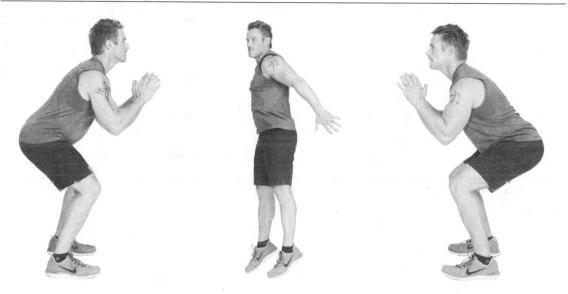

Setup: Stand with your feet hip-width apart and lower into a squat.

Action: Jump up, swinging your arms overhead, and rotate yourself 180 degrees to the right while in the air. Land with your knees bent and lower into a squat. Jump up, rotating 180 degrees to the left.

✱ *Jessie's Tip: If you aren't comfortable rotating 180 degrees, start with a 90-degree jump.*

■ Plank Jack (see page 145 for photos)

Setup: Assume a push-up position, arms extended, hands on the floor, and legs extended with feet together.

Action: Jump your feet out to the sides, then back together.

■ Switch Jump Lunge (see page 137 for photos)

Setup: Lunge forward with your right thigh parallel to the floor, your left leg back.

Action: Jump up and switch leg positions. Land in a lunge with your left foot forward. Repeat on the other side.

■ Russian Twist

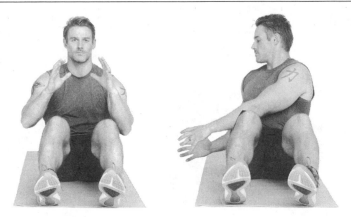

Setup: Sit on the floor with knees bent and heels about a foot from your hips. Lean back slightly to a 45-degree angle without rounding your back.

Action: Place arms in front of your chest, pull navel into your spine and rotate torso to the right, come back to center and rotate left.

FULL THROTTLE DAY 8: BUILD—STRENGTH TRAINING

■ Pull Day

Four sets of 15 reps
Recovery: 30–60 seconds between sets

■ Single Arm Row (see "Lunge with Single Arm Row," page 141 for photos)

Setup: Stand in a staggered stance with your left foot forward and right leg back. Holding a dumbbell in your right hand, bend at your hips and knees and lower your torso almost parallel to the floor. Extend your right arm.

Action: Pull the dumbbell up until your elbow passes your torso, keeping your elbow close to your side. Lower the dumbbells back to start position.

■ Biceps Curl (see page 111 for photos)

Setup: Stand with your feet shoulder-width apart with a dumbbell in each hand, palms facing forward, arms hanging down at your sides.

Action: Keeping your elbows close to your torso, curl the dumbbells up toward your shoulders. Return to start position.

■ Single Leg Dead Lift

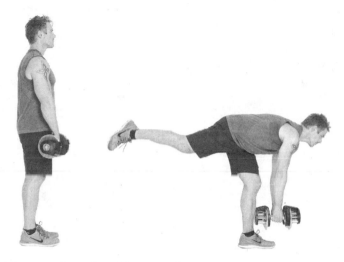

Setup: Start with your feet shoulder-width apart, toes pointing straight ahead. Hold a pair of dumbbells in front of your thighs with your palms facing your body.

Action: Lift your left leg a few inches off the floor, then lower the dumbbells toward the floor as you raise your left leg behind you. Keep your back straight and your right knee slightly bent. Return to starting position. Complete all reps on the right side, then switch sides.

■ Resistance Band Row (see page 112 for photos)

Setup: Attach the resistance band door attachment at chest height. Stand facing the door, holding both handles and with your knees slightly bent.

Action: Reach forward with your arms in line with your shoulders. Pull the band back until your elbows pass your torso. Return to start.

■ Lat Pullover

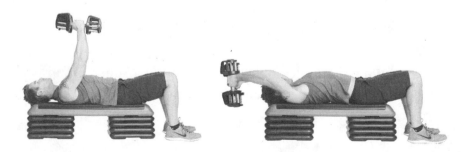

Setup: Lie down on a bench or mat. Hold a dumbbell in each hand over your chest, keeping your elbows slightly bent.

Action: Extend your arms over your chest, palms facing in. Keeping your elbows slightly bent, lower the dumbbells in an arc back over your head toward the floor. Bring your elbows level with your head, then return to start position.

✱ *Jessie's Tip: If you are using heavier weights, hold one heavy dumbbell with both hands.*

FULL THROTTLE DAY 9: BURN—METABOLIC TRAINING

◼ Five Exercises, 1 Minute Each Exercise, Repeat Circuit Three Times

Perform each exercise for 60 seconds, then move on to the next exercise. Complete one circuit, recover for 90 seconds, then repeat the circuit three times.

◼ Straddle Bench Jump

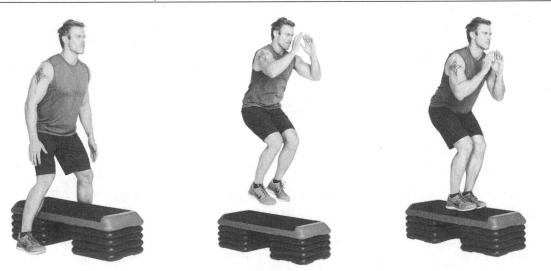

Setup: Stand on a bench with your knees slightly bent and your arms in front at shoulder height.

Action: Jump down to straddle the bench, landing in a squat. Jump back onto the bench, landing with your feet together and knees bent.

■ **Single Leg Dead Lift with Row**

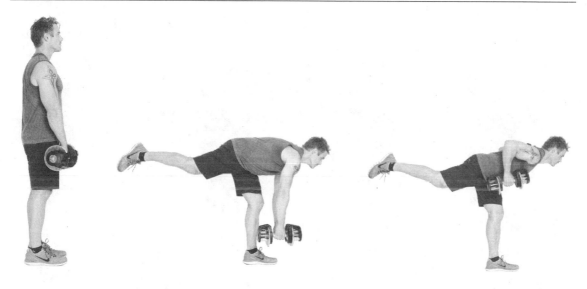

Setup: Start with your feet shoulder-width apart, toes pointing straight ahead. Hold a pair of dumbbells in front of your thighs with your palms facing your body.

Action: Lift your left leg a few inches off the floor, then lower the dumbbells toward the floor as you raise your left leg behind you. Keep your back straight and your right knee slightly bent. Pull the dumbbells up toward your torso. Return to starting position. Repeat for 30 seconds on the right side, then switch sides.

■ **Forward Lunge with Biceps Curl** (see page 147 for photos)

Setup: Stand with your feet hip-width apart, holding a dumbbell in each hand, arms down at your side, palms facing in.

Action: Take a step forward with your right foot and bend your right knee to 90 degrees, simultaneously curling the dumbbells up toward your shoulders. Push off your right foot and return to starting position. Complete all reps on the right side, then switch sides.

■ Curtsy, Lunge, Squat on Bench

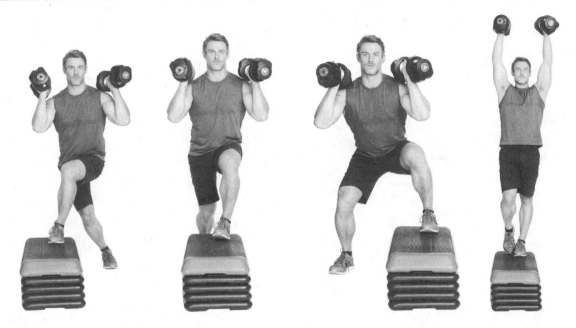

Setup: Stand behind the narrow end of a bench with a dumbbell in each hand. Step your right foot onto the bench, step your left leg behind you and to the right so your thighs cross, bend both knees, and keep your hips pointing forward.

Action: Press off your left foot and lunge behind the bench. Press off your left foot again and step into a squat. Keeping your right foot on the bench, press down with your right foot to lift your left leg onto the bench. Repeat all reps on the right side, then switch sides.

■ Plank Knee Cross (see "Plank with Alternating Knee Cross," page 130 for photos)

Setup: Start in a plank position with your hands under your shoulders.

Action: Bring your right knee toward your left elbow. Return to start position and repeat with your left leg.

FULL THROTTLE DAY 10: BUILD—STRENGTH TRAINING

■ Leg Day

Four sets of 15 reps
Recovery: 30–60 seconds between sets

■ Curtsy, Lunge, Squat on Bench (see page 170 for photos)

Setup: Stand behind the narrow end of a bench with a dumbbell in each hand. Step your right foot onto the bench, step your left leg behind you and to the right so your thighs cross, bend both knees, and keep your hips pointing forward.

Action: Press off your left foot and lunge behind the bench. Press off your left foot again and step into a squat. Keeping your right foot on the bench, press down with your right foot to lift your left leg onto the bench. Repeat all reps on the right side, then switch sides.

■ Dead Lift (see page 57 for photos)

Setup: Start with your feet shoulder-width apart, toes pointing straight ahead. Hold a pair of dumbbells in front of your thighs with your palms facing your body.

Action: Keeping your back straight, hinge forward at your hips and lower your torso until it's almost parallel to the floor. Lower the dumbbells toward your feet. Squeeze your glutes and push your hips forward to return to standing.

■ Single Leg Glute Bridge on Bench

Setup: Lie on the floor with your feet on the bench, arms by your sides, and knees bent to 90 degrees.

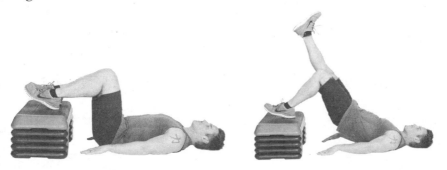

Action: Press through your left heel and lift your right leg and your hips up, squeezing your glutes at the top. Slowly return to starting position.

■ Pistol Squat (see page 162 for photos)

Setup: Stand on your right foot with your left leg extended in front of you.

Action: Bend your right knee and squat down as far as you can while keeping your left leg lifted. Extend your right leg to return to start position.

■ Pulse Squat

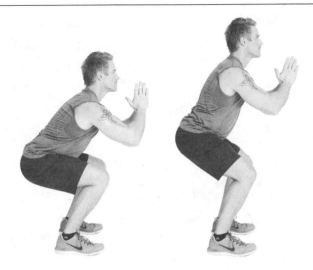

Setup: Stand with your feet hip-width apart, arms at your sides.

Action: Bend your knees like you're sitting in a chair until your thighs are nearly parallel to the floor. Hold the squat position and pulse a few inches up and down 15 times.

FULL THROTTLE DAY 11: BURN—ATHLETIC TRAINING

20 seconds work, 10 seconds recovery

Repeat one exercise four times for 20 seconds on, then 10 seconds rest.

Recover 30–60 seconds before moving on to the next exercise. 4 × 20 working, 10 seconds recovery

Up to 60 seconds rest

■ Squat Thrust (see page 93 for photos)

Setup: Stand with your feet together, arms at your sides.

Action: Bend your knees and place your palms on the floor with your arms on the outside of your knees. Shift your weight onto your palms. Jump both feet back and land in plank position. Jump both feet forward and return to standing.

■ Jump Forward, Jog Back (see page 144 for photos)

Setup: Start standing with your feet shoulder-width apart, knees slightly bent.

Action: Imagine there is a cone 3 feet in front of you. Squat down and jump forward toward the cone. Jog back to starting position.

■ Mountain Climber (see page 136 for photos)

Setup: Assume a push-up position, arms extended, and hands on the floor, legs extended.

Action: Keeping your body in a straight line, bring your right knee toward your chest. Return to start and repeat with your left leg.

■ Pass the Ball, Shoot the Ball (see page 90 for photos)

Setup: Stand with your feet slightly wider than hip-width apart, knees slightly bent and hands at chest level.

Action: Imagine you are holding a basketball at your chest. Pivot to your right side and push your arms out as if passing the ball. Come back to starting position and jump up or lift up on your toes and pretend to shoot the ball. Repeat on the other side.

■ Plank Knee Cross (see "Plank with Alternating Knee Cross," page 130 for photos)

Setup: Start in a plank position with your hands under your shoulders.

Action: Bring your right knee toward your left elbow. Return to start position and repeat with your left leg.

■ High Knee Sprint (see page 93 for photos)

Setup: Stand with feet hip-width apart, knees slightly bent, and arms at your sides.

Action: Bring your right knee up to hip level, left arm reaching toward the ceiling, push off your left foot and switch legs and arms bringing your left leg up to hip level and right arm toward the ceiling.

FULL THROTTLE DAY 12: BUILD—STRENGTH TRAINING

■ Full Body

Four sets of 16 reps
Recovery: 30–60 seconds between sets

■ Renegade Row (see page 160 for photos)

Setup: Assume the push-up position with your arms straight, feet slightly wider than shoulder-width, and hands holding a pair of dumbbells directly under your shoulders.

Action: Lift your left elbow toward the ceiling until your elbow passes your torso. Lower the weight, and repeat on the other side. Each row is counted as one rep.

■ Lunge with Overhead Press

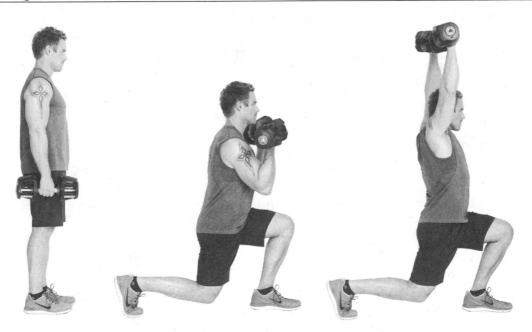

Setup: Stand with feet shoulder-width apart holding a dumbbell in each hand, arms hanging at your sides, palms facing each other.

Action: Curl dumbbells up to your shoulders as you step your right foot forward into lunge. Press dumbbells overhead, then press into your right heel to return to standing.

■ Chest Fly Lat Pullover on Stability Ball

Setup: Sit on the stability ball, holding a dumbbell in each hand, dumbbells on your thighs. Slowly walk your feet forward and slide your torso down the ball until your head, shoulders, and upper back are on the ball. Your feet should be parallel and your knees

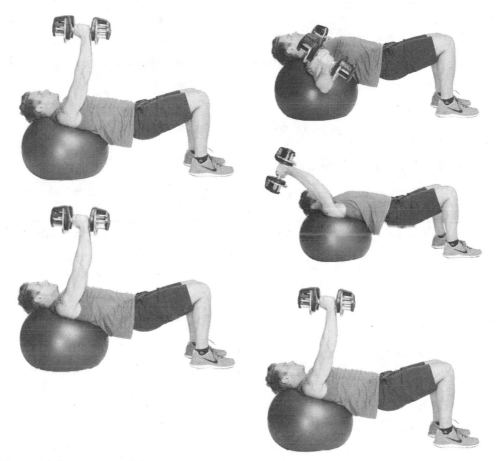

shoulder-width apart and bent 90 degrees so your thighs and torso are parallel with the floor.

Action: Position the dumbbells over your chest with your palms facing each other. Press the dumbbells upward above your chest, elbows straight but not locked. Lower the dumbbells until they are level with your chest. Press the dumbbells back to starting position, lower the dumbbells behind your head, then bring the dumbbells over your chest. One rep is one chest fly and one lat pullover.

■ Stability Ball Back Extension (see page 101 for photos)

Setup: Lie facedown on a stability ball with your hands on the ball at your sides, about 6 inches apart. Press your feet against a wall or sturdy object.

Action: Lift your torso up until your body forms a straight line.

* *Jessie's Tip: To make it more challenging, place your hands behind your head.*

■ Sumo Squat Biceps Curl (see page 105 for photos)

Setup: Stand with your feet slightly wider than hip-width apart, toes out, holding a dumbbell in each hand, palms facing forward.

Action: Bend your knees and lower your body until your thighs are parallel to the floor. Push yourself back up as you curl the dumbbells to your shoulders.

FULL THROTTLE DAY 13: SLOW BURN AND FLOW

Try to jog continuously for 30 minutes today. You are not sprinting, so don't worry about your pace at all. You want a comfortable, easy jog on relatively flat terrain. If you feel breathless after 10 or 15 minutes, slow down to a brisk walk until you are completely recovered, then resume jogging. Alternate between brisk walking and jogging at any point, as many times as you feel comfortable, but try to move continuously for 30 minutes.

PART 2: FLOW

■ Downward-Facing Dog (see page 95 for photos)

Setup: Begin in a plank position. As you inhale, spread your fingers wide and press both palms firmly into the mat while simultaneously tucking your toes under. As you exhale, begin to draw your hips toward the ceiling, making the shape of an inverted V. Your head and neck should be between your upper arms. Bend your knees as much as you need to while maintaining equal weight on your hands and feet. Hold for three to five breath cycles.

Flow from Downward-Facing Dog into Low Lunge.

■ Low Lunge (see page 96 for photos)

Step your right foot between your hands, coming into a low lunge position. Shift your weight forward slightly to allow your right thigh to become parallel to the floor while remaining on the ball of you back foot (that should be your left foot).

Flow from Low Lunge into Warrior I.

■ Warrior I (see page 96 for photos)

Keeping your front foot facing forward, turn your back foot slightly outward and let your back foot rest flat at a 45-degree angle. Reach your arms overhead so they are parallel to one another. Your hips should still be facing forward as you lower your shoulders away from your ears and lift your core as you bend your front knee (your right knee) into a 90-degree angle. Hold this position for three to five breath cycles.

Flow from Warrior I into Warrior II.

■ Warrior II (see page 97 for photos)

Rotate your weight to the left and bring your arms straight out to your sides, parallel to the floor. Although the position of your feet does not change, your hips should now face the left. Your front leg (your right leg) should be bent while your back (left leg) is straight. This is Warrior II pose. Hold it for three to five breath cycles.

Flow from Warrior II into Side Angle.

■ Side Angle (see page 97 for photos)

Drop your right forearm on your right thigh and tilt your torso open, so that your left hand is now up in the air, reaching for the ceiling. Hold for three to five breath cycles.

Repeat this sequence on the other side. This means that you'll step back with your right leg back into Downward Facing Dog and repeat the entire flow on your left side.

Continue to alternate sets between sides two to five times.

FULL THROTTLE DAY 14: BUILD—STRENGTH TRAINING

■ Push Day

Four sets of 15 reps
Recovery: 30–60 seconds between sets

■ Stability Ball Push-up (see page 140 for photos)

Setup: Come into a plank position, with your toes or shins resting on the ball. Place your hands shoulder-width apart.

Action: Bend your elbows to a 90-degree angle, then press back to starting position.

■ Pistol Squat (see page 162 for photos)

Setup: Stand on your right foot with your left leg extended in front of you.

Action: Bend your right knee and squat down as far as you can while keeping your left leg lifted. Extend your right leg to return to start position.

■ Chest Press on Bench (see page 162 for photos)

Setup: Lie on a bench with a dumbbell in each hand and your feet flat on the floor. Position the dumbbells over your chest with your palms facing forward.

Action: Press the dumbbells upward above your chest, elbows straight but not locked. Lower the dumbbells until they are level with your chest. Return to starting position.

■ Lying Triceps Extension on the Bench (see page 163 for photos)

Setup: Lie on a bench, holding a dumbbell in each hand. Extend your arms to a 90-degree angle from the floor.

Action: Bend your elbows so your forearms are parallel to the floor. Straighten your arms without locking your elbows.

■ Front Raise/Lateral Raise (see page 163 for photos)

Setup: Stand with your feet shoulder-width apart, holding a dumbbell in each hand, palms facing each other.

Action: Keeping your elbows slightly bent, raise the dumbbells to the sides until your arms are parallel with the floor. Lower to start position. Turn your hands so your palms face your thighs, and raise the dumbbells forward until they are parallel to the floor. One front and one lateral raise are counted as one repetition.

FULL THROTTLE DAY 15: BURN—ATHLETIC TRAINING

■ Tabata Training

20 seconds work, 10 seconds recovery
Repeat one exercise four times for 20 seconds on, then 10 seconds rest.
Recover 30–60 seconds before moving on to the next exercise.

■ Speed Skate (see page 91 for photos)

Setup: Stand with your feet hip-width apart, knees slightly bent.

Action: Leap to the right side and land on your right leg, reaching down with your left hand toward your right knee or toes. Leap to the left side and land on your left leg, reaching down with your right hand toward your left knee or toes.

■ Spiderman Push-up (see page 164 for photos)

Setup: Start in a plank position with your hands under your shoulders.

Action: Bring your right knee outward toward your right elbow. Return to start position and repeat with left leg.

■ 180-Degree Jump (see page 165 for photos)

Setup: Stand with your feet hip-width apart and lower into a squat.

Action: Jump up, swinging your arms overhead, and rotate yourself 180 degrees to the right while in the air. Land with your knees bent and lower into a squat. Jump up, rotating 180 degrees to the left.

✳ *Jessie's Tip: If you aren't comfortable rotating 180 degrees, start with a 90-degree jump.*

■ Plank Jack (see page 145 for photos)

Setup: Assume a push-up position, arms extended, hands on the floor, and legs extended with feet together.

Action: Jump your feet out to the sides, then back together.

■ Switch Jump Lunge (see page 137 for photos)

Setup: Lunge forward with your right thigh parallel to the floor, your left leg back.

Action: Jump up and switch leg positions. Land in a lunge with your left foot forward. Repeat on the other side.

■ Russian Twist (see page 166 for photos)

Setup: Sit on the floor with knees bent and heels about a foot from your hips. Lean back slightly to a 45-degree angle without rounding your back.

Action: Place arms in front of your chest, pull navel into your spine and rotate torso to the right, come back to center and rotate left.

FULL THROTTLE DAY 16: BUILD—STRENGTH TRAINING

■ Pull Day

Four sets of 15 reps
Recovery: 30–60 seconds between sets

■ Single Arm Row (see "Lunge with Single Arm Row," page 141 for photos)

Setup: Stand in a staggered stance with your left foot forward and right leg back. Holding a dumbbell in your right hand, bend at your hips and knees and lower your torso almost parallel to the floor. Extend your right arm.

Action: Pull the dumbbell up until your elbow passes your torso, keeping your elbow close to your side. Lower the dumbbells back to start position.

■ Biceps Curl (see page 111 for photos)

Setup: Stand with your feet shoulder-width apart with a dumbbell in each hand, palms facing forward, arms hanging down at your sides.

Action: Keeping your elbows close to your torso, curl the dumbbells up toward your shoulders. Return to start position.

■ Single Leg Dead Lift (see page 167 for photos)

Setup: Start with your feet shoulder-width apart, toes pointing straight ahead. Hold a pair of dumbbells in front of your thighs with your palms facing your body.

Action: Lift your left leg a few inches off the floor, and lower the dumbbells toward the floor as you raise your left leg behind you. Keep your back straight and your right knee slightly bent. Return to starting position. Complete all reps on the right side, then switch sides.

■ Resistance Band Row (see page 112 for photos)

Setup: Attach the resistance band door attachment at chest height. Stand facing the door, holding both handles and with your knees slightly bent.

Action: Reach forward with your arms in line with your shoulders. Pull the band back until your elbows pass your torso. Return to start.

■ Lat Pullover (see page 111 for photos)

Setup: Lie faceup on a bench or mat. Hold a dumbbell in each hand over your chest, keeping your elbows slightly bent.

Action: Extend your arms over your chest, palms facing in. Keeping your elbows slightly bent, lower the dumbbells in an arc back over your head toward the floor. Raise the dumbbells back over the chest.

✻ *Jessie's Tip: If you are using heavier weights, hold one heavy dumbbell with both hands.*

FULL THROTTLE DAY 17: BURN—METABOLIC TRAINING

■ Five Exercises, 1 Minute Each Exercise, Repeat Circuit Three Times

Perform each exercise for 60 seconds, then move on to the next exercise. Complete one circuit, recover for 90 seconds, then repeat the circuit three times.

■ Renegade Row (see page 160 for photos)

Setup: Assume the push-up position with your arms straight, feet slightly wider than shoulder-width, and hands holding a pair of dumbbells directly under your shoulders.

Action: Lift your left elbow toward the ceiling until your elbow passes your torso. Lower the weight, and repeat on the other side. Each row is counted as one rep.

■ Squat Jump (see page 146 for photos)

Setup: Stand with your feet shoulder-width apart, arms at your sides. Sit back into a squat until your thighs are parallel to the floor.

Action: Jump up explosively. Land with bent knees.

■ Stability Ball Push-up and Pike (see pages 140 and 100 for photos)

Setup: Start with your torso on the ball and hands and feet on the floor. Walk your hands forward until your legs are straight and your toes are on top of the ball. Hands are under shoulders.

Action: Lower yourself until your chest almost touches the floor. Press your upper body back to starting position. Keeping your legs straight, pull your feet toward your chest and push your hips toward the ceiling as the ball rolls in. Continue until your hips are directly under your shoulders. Slowly lower back to starting position. Continue alternating one push-up and one pike.

■ Jump Forward, Jog Back (see page 144 for photos)

Setup: Start standing with your feet shoulder-width apart, knees slightly bent.

Action: Imagine there is a cone 3 feet in front of you. Squat down and jump forward toward the cone. Jog back to starting position.

■ V Sit with Incline Dumbbell Chest Press (see page 161 for photos)

Setup: Sit on the floor with your feet flat, holding a light dumbbell in each hand in front of your shoulders. Lean back so your torso is at a 45-degree angle.

Action: Engage your core and press the dumbbells away from your body until your arms are straight. Return to start.

FULL THROTTLE DAY 18: BUILD—STRENGTH TRAINING

■ Leg Day

Four sets of 15 reps
Recovery: 30–60 seconds between sets

■ Curtsy, Lunge, Squat on Bench (see page 170 for photos)

Setup: Stand behind the narrow end of a bench with a dumbbell in each hand. Step your right foot onto the bench, step your left leg behind you and to the right so your thighs cross, bend both knees, and keep your hips pointing forward.

Action: Press off your left foot and lunge behind the bench. Press off your left foot again and step into a squat. Keeping your right foot on the bench, press down with your right foot to lift your left leg onto the bench. Repeat all reps on the right side, then switch sides.

■ Dead Lift (see page 57 for photos)

Setup: Start with your feet shoulder-width apart, toes pointing straight ahead. Hold a pair of dumbbells in front of your thighs with palms your facing your body.

Action: Keeping your back straight, hinge forward at your hips and lower your torso until it's almost parallel with the floor. Lower the dumbbells toward your feet. Squeeze your glutes and push your hips forward to return to standing.

■ Single Leg Glute Bridge on Bench (see page 171 for photos)

Setup: Lie on the floor with your feet on the bench, arms by your sides, and knees bent to 90 degrees.

Action: Press through your left heel and lift your right leg and your hips up, squeezing your glutes at the top. Slowly return to starting position.

■ Pistol Squat (see page 162 for photos)

Setup: Stand on your right foot with your left leg extended in front of you.

Action: Bend your right knee and squat down as far as you can while keeping your left leg lifted. Extend your right leg to return to start position.

■ Pulse Squat (see page 172 for photos)

Setup: Stand with your feet hip-width apart, arms at your sides.

Action: Bend your knees like you're sitting in a chair until your thighs are nearly parallel to the floor. Hold the squat position and pulse a few inches up and down 15 times.

FULL THROTTLE DAY 19: BURN—ATHLETIC TRAINING

4 × 20 working, 10 seconds recovery
Up to 60 seconds rest

■ Squat Thrust (see page 93 for photos)

Setup: Stand with your feet together, arms at your sides.

Action: Bend your knees and place your palms on the floor with your arms on the outside of your knees. Shift your weight onto your palms. Jump both feet back and land in plank position. Jump both feet forward and return to standing.

■ Jump Forward, Jog Back (see page 144 for photos)

Setup: Start standing with your feet shoulder-width apart, knees slightly bent.

Action: Imagine there is a cone 3 feet in front of you. Squat down and jump forward toward the cone. Jog back to starting position.

■ Mountain Climber (see page 136 for photos)

Setup: Assume a push-up position, arms extended, hands on the floor, legs extended.

Action: Keeping your body in a straight line, bring your right knee toward your chest. Return to start and repeat with your left leg.

■ Pass the Ball, Shoot the Ball (see page 90 for photos)

Setup: Stand with your feet slightly wider than hip-width apart, knees slightly bent and hands at chest level.

Action: Imagine you are holding a basketball at your chest. Pivot to your right side and push your arms out as if passing the ball. Come back to starting position and jump up or lift up on your toes and pretend to shoot the ball. Repeat on the other side.

■ Plank Knee Cross (see "Plank with Alternating Knee Cross," page 130 for photos)

Setup: Start in a plank position with your hands under your shoulders.

Action: Bring your right knee toward your left elbow. Return to start position and repeat with your left leg.

■ High Knee Sprint (see page 93 for photos)

Setup: Stand with feet hip-width apart, knees slightly bent, and arms at your sides.

Action: Bring your right knee up to hip level, left arm reaching toward the ceiling, push off your left foot and switch legs and arms bringing your left leg up to hip level and right arm toward the ceiling.

FULL THROTTLE DAY 20: BUILD—STRENGTH TRAINING

■ Full Body

Four sets of 16 reps
Recovery: 30–60 seconds between sets

■ Renegade Row (see page 160 for photos)

Setup: Assume the push-up position with your arms straight, feet slightly wider than shoulder-width, and hands holding a pair of dumbbells directly under your shoulders.

Action: Lift your left elbow toward the ceiling until your elbow passes your torso. Lower the weight, and repeat on the other side. Each row is counted as one rep.

■ Lunge with Overhead Press (see page 174 for photos)

Setup: Stand with feet shoulder-width apart holding a dumbbell in each hand, arms hanging at your sides palms facing each other.

Action: Curl dumbbells up to your shoulders as you step your right foot forward into lunge. Press dumbbells overhead, then press into your right heel to return to standing.

▪ Chest Fly Lat Pullover on Stability Ball (see page 175 for photos)

Setup: Sit on the stability ball, holding a dumbbell in each hand, dumbbells on your thighs. Slowly walk your feet forward and slide your torso down the ball until your head, shoulders, and upper back are on the ball. Feet should be parallel and knees shoulder-width apart and bent 90 degrees so your thighs and torso are parallel with the floor.

Action: Position the dumbbells over your chest, palms facing each other. Press the dumbbells upward above your chest, elbows straight but not locked. Lower the dumbbells until they are level with your chest. Press the dumbbells back to starting position, lower the dumbbells behind your head, then bring the dumbbells over your chest. One rep is one chest fly and one lat pullover.

▪ Stability Ball Back Extension (see page 101 for photos)

Setup: Lie facedown on a stability ball with your hands on the ball at your sides, about 6 inches apart. Press your feet against a wall or sturdy object.

Action: Lift your torso up until your body forms a straight line.

* *Jessie's Tip: To make it more challenging, perform the exercise with your fingertips by your ears instead of on the ball.*

▪ Sumo Squat Biceps Curl (see page 105 for photos)

Setup: Stand with your feet slightly wider than hip-width apart, toes out, holding a dumbbell in each hand, palms facing inward.

Action: Bend your knees and lower your body until thighs are parallel to the floor. Push yourself back up as you rotate your wrists outward and curl the dumbbells to your shoulders.

FULL THROTTLE DAY 21: BURN—METABOLIC TRAINING

▪ Five Exercises, 1 Minute Each Exercise, Repeat Circuit Three Times

Perform each exercise for 60 seconds, then move on to the next exercise. Complete one circuit, recover for 90 seconds, then repeat the circuit three times.

■ **Straddle Bench Jump** (see page 168 for photos)

Setup: Stand on a bench with your knees slightly bent and your arms in front at shoulder height.

Action: Jump down to straddle the bench, landing in a squat. Jump back onto the bench, landing with your feet together and knees bent.

■ **Single Leg Dead Lift with Row** (see page 169 for photos)

Setup: Start with your feet shoulder-width apart, toes pointing straight ahead. Hold a pair of dumbbells in front of your thighs with your palms facing your body.

Action: Lift your left leg a few inches off the floor, then lower the dumbbells toward the floor as you raise your left leg behind you. Keep your back straight and your right knee slightly bent, and pull the dumbbells up toward your torso. Return to starting position. Repeat for 30 seconds on the right side, then switch sides.

■ **Forward Lunge with Biceps Curl** (see page 147 for photos)

Setup: Stand with your feet hip-width apart, holding a dumbbell in each hand, arms down at your side, palms facing in.

Action: Take a step forward with your right foot and bend your right knee to 90 degrees, simultaneously curling the dumbbells up toward your shoulders. Push off your right foot and return to starting position. Complete all reps on the right side, then switch sides.

■ **Curtsy, Lunge, Squat on Bench** (see page 170 for photos)

Setup: Stand behind the narrow end of a bench with a dumbbell in each hand. Step your right foot onto the bench, step your left leg behind you and to the right so your thighs cross, bend both knees, and keep your hips pointing forward.

Action: Press off your left foot and lunge behind the bench. Press off your left foot again and step into a squat. Keeping your right foot on the bench, press down with your right foot to lift your left leg onto the bench. Repeat all reps on the right side, then switch sides.

■ **Plank Knee Cross** (see "Plank with Alternating Knee Cross," page 130 for photos)

Setup: Start in a plank position with your hands under your shoulders.

Action: Bring your right knee toward your left elbow. Return to start position and repeat with your left leg.

WEEKEND WARRIOR WORKOUT CHALLENGE

How many can you do? Challenge yourself by repeating exercises from each style of training (strength, athletic, metabolic) at your appropriate level with more intensity and more repetitions than usual! Perform each exercise set once, take a 30–60 second recovery, then move on to the next exercise in the sequence. Once you have finished set 4, take a 2-minute break if you need it, then repeat the entire sequence as many times as you can (taking the 60-second rest between sets and the 2-minute break after the fourth set). Record your results and try it again when you are well rested next week and up for a challenge!

Set 1

Strength Training (Push)
Knee Push-up
Athletic Training
Pass the Ball, Shoot the Ball
Metabolic Training
Squat with Dumbbell Overall Press

Set 2

Strength Training (Pull)
Dumbbell Row
Athletic Training
Side Shuffle
Metabolic Training
Alternating Step-up

Set 3

Strength Training (Legs)
Squat
Athletic Training
Lunge Kick Lunge
Metabolic Training
Sumo Squat Biceps Curl

Set 4

Strength Training (Full Body)
Squat Knee Raise
Athletic Training
Alternating Elbow to Knee
Metabolic Training
Reverse Lunge Lateral Raise

BONUS WEEKEND YOGA WORKOUT

Setup: Take a moment to sit cross-legged. Let your thoughts go, release your "to-do" list and anything you may have been stressed out about lately. This is your time. This is your space. Take it, and reap the benefits of a calmer, more energized day after your practice. Take five deep breaths. On the in breath say silently in your head: Acceptance. On the out breath say: Peace.

Action:

■ Stretch

Stand up and reach your arms high above your head, stretching your ribs up and taking two deep breaths. Bend over to your right, keeping your shoulders dropped even though your arms are above your head. Next bend to your left, allowing your right side to stretch out and elongate now. Come back to standing straight and drop your arms.

Now stretch your arms up once more and immediately dive forward, bending at the waist until you're hanging over your legs, only as deeply as your body wants to go today. Make sure you release your head and tension in your neck. Let the tension melt off you like snow melting off a tree in the sun.

■ Downward Facing Dog

Come into Downward Facing Dog. You've held this pose during The Program as part of your flow workout, but this time you are leaning down into it from the stretch, rather than rising into it from a plank. Bend your legs and plant your hands on the ground, shoulder-width apart. Keep your feet about shoulder-width apart, legs as straight as possible, and bring the hips up high while keeping your back straight and hinging at the waist. Your palms are planted firmly on the ground, you look sort of like a tent. Your head and neck should be between your upper arms. Bend your knees as much as you need to while maintaining equal weight on your hands and feet. Hold for three to five breath cycles, releasing a little more tension on each breath out and sinking into the pose.

■ Plank and Chaturanga Hold

Come into plank position (or the upper part of a push up) and hold it for five breaths. Now, slowly lower yourself down, elbows tight against your body, without touching the floor, and hold hovering like this for one or two breaths. This lower push-up position is called "chaturanga" in yoga. Next, release and lie on the floor on your stomach for two breaths. Now get back into upper plank position, hold for five breaths again, lower down into chaturanga (that lower push-up position, ensuring your butt is low and in line with your shoulders as much as possible). Keep a straight back, just like a regular plank. It's not easy! This is a great core and arm and leg workout. Hold it for three breaths this time. Lower down and then take Upward Facing Dog (arch your back up, look up to the sky shoulders dropped, and keep your hips and legs on the ground) for three to five breaths.

▪ Side Plank

From the floor or standing come into Downward Facing Dog.

Now switch onto your right foot and right hand only, stacking your left foot, looking out to the side and holding Side Plank. Keep your body in a straight line. Hold for four breaths. Come back to Downward Facing Dog, and switch over to the other side-facing plank. Hold 4 breaths. Keep your core tight through all poses and transitions—breathe while you move and hold!

Back to Downward Facing Dog. Walk or jump your feet in until you're hanging over your legs, then roll up one vertebra at a time to standing. Ground your feet and shake off any tension.

▪ Chair Pose

Squat while sticking your butt out, holding your back and neck long and straight, until you are in Chair Pose. Reach your arms over your head parallel to your shoulders. Reach even as you hold your squat. Stay in this position for five breaths. Come to standing.

▪ Squat Work

Take 15 deep squats with your hands on your hips and straighten while breathing deeply. At the top (when you're standing tall), squeeze your butt and at the low point of the squat (when you're sitting) stick your butt out like you're sitting on a chair. Keep your back straight, core tight, shoulders dropped. You'll feel this in your glutes!

▪ Tree Balance Pose

Bring one foot up until the flat of your foot is against the inside of your standing leg. Stand straight and balance on one foot by engaging your core. Lift your hands above your head and touch your palms together. Hold as long as you can! Can you hold it for about six breaths? Breathe deeply! You are learning to stay balanced, while clearing your mind and strengthening your core muscles.

■ Closing Meditation

Come back to standing, bring your hands together in prayer in front of your chest. Take some deep breaths with your eyes closed, simply do nothing and feel your breath in your body as you learn to be present and accept yourself. Next silently thank yourself for taking this time to honor your body and health. Sending gratitude to your body and self will increase your acceptance and help strengthen your resolve to make healthy choices for your diet, exercise, and life. It's like giving you inner fortitude toward your will power!

The Recipes

I'm a pretty basic cook, and so are most of the recipes that follow. The food exchange lists and the nutrition information provided in the meal plan day charts can help you make swaps from meal to meal if you feel like making something different but want to stick to your PCF ratio. I threw in a few of my favorite scrambles and salads, which aren't called for on any specific day, but you might want to try them as you move forward. If you want to follow the meal plan strictly, most meals have a recipe provided, but the snacks and a few of the dinners are so straightforward they do not need one (I assume you already have your own preferred method of grilling flank steak or poaching salmon, for example).

Many people find that as they move more, they are hungrier and food just plain tastes better. Take advantage of this if it happens to you on The Program, and use the opportunity to find new ingredients you love and healthy foods that make you feel great.

Nutrition information calculated with ESHA, The Food Processor Nutrition Analysis and Fitness Software, 2005.

Avocado Egg White Bake (Build Day 14)

If you hard-boil a few eggs when you have 15 minutes and put them in your refrigerator, it'll save you a step when you make this and you'll have high-protein snacks ready and waiting.

½ large avocado, pit removed
2 egg whites
Salt and pepper, to taste
1 cup chopped honeydew melon, on side
1 hard-boiled egg, on side

Directions:

Preheat oven to 425 degrees. Using a spoon, hollow out the avocado half until there is approximately ½ inch of avocado meat remaining. Put the egg whites into the avocado half.

Bake the avocado half for about 15 minutes or to desired doneness. Top with salt and pepper.

Serve with the honeydew and hard-boiled egg on the side.

NUTRITION (with hard-boiled egg and honeydew melon, per meal plan): 290 calories, 16 g fat, 3 g sat fat, 21 g carbs, 6 g fiber, 16 g sugar, 15 g protein
EXCHANGES: 2 protein, 1 fruit, 2+ fats

Baked Egg "Muffins"

2 whole eggs
1 egg white
2 tablespoons thinly sliced scallion
2 tablespoons chopped red bell pepper
2 tablespoons shredded low-fat cheddar cheese
Salt and pepper, to taste
1 orange, on side

Directions:

Preheat oven to 350 degrees. Combine all ingredients except the orange in a medium bowl and whisk until combined.

Place the mixture into a small ramekin or one compartment of a muffin pan coated with cooking spray. Bake for 10–12 minutes or until the mixture is set.

Serve with the orange on the side.

NUTRITION (with small orange, per meal plan): 260 calories, 11 g fat, 4 g sat fat, 19 g carbs, 4 g fiber, 14 g sugar, 21 g protein
EXCHANGES: ½ dairy, 2½ protein, 1 fruit, ¼ vegetable, 2 fats

Black Bean Soup with Pico de Gallo (Cleanse)

This serves eight, with approximately 1½ cups per serving. If you're making it on a non-Cleanse day or for other family members who aren't doing the Cleanse portion of The Program, this soup tastes great with grilled skirt steak or grilled marinated chicken as an added protein option.

SOUP:

1 pound dry black beans (no presoaking necessary)
2 tomatoes, chopped
1 jalapeño pepper, sliced
½ small red onion, chopped
½ small bunch of cilantro, lightly chopped
1 tablespoon olive oil
4 cups vegetable stock
Kosher salt, to taste

GARNISH:

2 tomatoes, deseeded and chopped into small dice
½ jalapeño pepper, deseeded and minced
½ small bunch of cilantro, finely chopped
2 tablespoons red onion, minced
1 lemon, juiced
Kosher salt, to taste

Directions:

FOR THE SOUP:

Cook the black beans submerged in water for approximately 1 hour until tender. Strain the excess water and set the beans aside. In a large soup pot, sauté the tomato, jalapeño, onion, and cilantro in the olive oil for about 5 minutes. Add the cooked black beans, vegetable stock, and 1 cup water, and let simmer for 30 minutes. Transfer the soup in batches to a blender and puree until smooth. You do not need to strain the soup. Season with salt to taste.

FOR THE GARNISH:

Mix all ingredients in a medium bowl.

NUTRITION: 220 calories, 2½ g fat, 40 g carbs, 14 g fiber, 10 g sugar, 13 g protein
EXCHANGES: 1½ starch, 2 vegetables, ½ fat, 2 protein

Blueberry Chia Power Protein Pudding (Build Day 16)

This one is super easy, but you have to do it the night before, so plan ahead. It'll save you time in the morning!

- 2 tablespoons chia seeds
- 1 cup fat-free or reduced-fat milk
- 1 stevia packet
- 1 scoop protein powder
- 1 teaspoon ground cinnamon
- ½ cup blueberries

Directions:

Mix together chia seeds, milk, stevia, and protein powder. Allow the mixture to sit in the refrigerator for at least 8 hours. Top with the cinnamon and blueberries when you're ready to eat and enjoy.

NUTRITION: 370 calories, 10 g fat, 2.5 g sat fat, 39 g carbs, 11 g fiber, 22 g sugar, 32 g protein
EXCHANGES: 1 dairy, 3 protein, ½ fruit, 2 fats

Breakfast Burrito (Burn Day 17)

- 1 teaspoon canola oil
- ½ cup bell peppers
- ½ cup onion
- 1 whole egg
- 2 egg white
- 1 8-inch whole wheat tortilla
- 2 tablespoons shredded reduced-fat cheddar cheese
- 1 cup sliced strawberries, on side

Directions:

Heat the oil in a medium skillet over medium-high heat. Sauté the peppers and onions for about 8 minutes, until tender. Remove from the pan and set aside. Scramble the whole egg and egg whites, and cook to desired doneness. Place the scrambled eggs on the tortilla, and top with the cheese, peppers, and onions.

Serve with the strawberries on the side.

NUTRITION (with 1 cup sliced strawberries, per meal plan): 395 calories, 15 g fat, 3 g sat fat, 46 g carbs, 8 g fiber, 13 g sugar, 23 g protein
EXCHANGES: 1½ starches, 2 protein, ½ dairy, 1 fruit, 1 vegetables, 1 fat

Buffalo Chicken Salad (Build Day 12)

- 4–5 ounces grilled or roasted chicken breast, chopped or shredded, as you prefer
- 1 tablespoon hot sauce
- 2 cups chopped romaine
- ½ cup cooked quinoa
- ½ cup cherry tomatoes
- 2 tablespoons crumbled blue cheese
- 1 teaspoon olive oil
- 2 teaspoons apple cider vinegar
- 1 cup strawberries, on side

Directions:

Toss the cooked chicken with the hot sauce in a small bowl. Place the romaine in medium bowl, and top with the quinoa, chicken, tomatoes, and blue cheese. Drizzle with the oil and vinegar.

Serve with the strawberries on the side.

NUTRITION (with strawberries, per meal plan):
420 calories, 13 g fat, 3 g sat fat, 40 g carbs, 7 g fiber,
18 g sugar, 35 g protein
EXCHANGES: 1½ starch, ½ dairy, 4 protein, 1 fruit,
1½ vegetables, 1 fat

California Turkey Wrap (Burn Day 7)

2 ounces sliced turkey
1 ounce low-fat cheddar cheese
1 8-inch whole wheat tortilla
2 slices avocado
¼ cup chopped tomatoes
1 cup spring mix
1 cup raw carrots, on side
¼ cup Greek yogurt with dill, on side
1 cup chopped honeydew melon, on side

Directions:

Place the turkey and cheddar into tortilla and top with the avocado, tomatoes, and spring mix.

Serve with the carrots, yogurt dip, and honeydew on the side.

NUTRITION (with carrots and honeydew melon, per meal plan): 450 calories, 11 g fat, 3 g sat fat, 60 g carbs, 11 g fiber, 23 g sugar, 26 g protein
EXCHANGES: 1½ starches, 3 protein, 1 fruit, 2 vegetables, 1 fat, 1+ dairy

Carrot-Ginger Soup (Cleanse)

This soup serves eight, with approximately 1½ cups per serving. If you are not eating this during a Cleanse day, it would be delicious and pack more protein with the addition of a little seafood, such as seared scallops or lobster.

1 medium white onion, chopped (about 1 cup)
2 garlic cloves, minced
2 tablespoons peeled and sliced fresh ginger
1 teaspoon ground cumin
1 tablespoon olive oil
3 pounds carrots, peeled and chopped
8 cups vegetable stock
Kosher salt, to taste
Ground white pepper, to taste
1 cup broccoli, broken into small florets
1 teaspoon chopped chives per bowl of soup

Directions:

In a medium soup pot, sauté the onions, garlic, ginger, and cumin in the olive oil over medium heat. Add the carrots and continue to cook for 5 more minutes, stirring constantly. Pour in the vegetable stock and let simmer until the carrots become tender. Transfer the soup in batches to a blender and blend until smooth, adding salt and pepper to taste. Note: start the blender on low speed to avoid splattering. Optional: when soup is smooth and seasoned, pass through a fine-mesh strainer. Blanch the broccoli in boiling water for 5 minutes until bright green and stir into the soup.

Serve with the chopped chives on top.

NUTRITION: 128 calories, 2.4 g fat, 25 g carbs, 6 g fiber, 9 g sugar, 2 g protein
EXCHANGES: 3 vegetables, ½ fat

Chicken, Bean, Rice, and Avocado Bowl (Burn Day 15)

3 ounces sliced, cooked chicken breast
1 cup chopped steamed broccoli
⅓ cup canned black beans, rinsed and drained
⅓ cup cooked brown rice
2 slices avocado
Hot sauce, to taste
2 kiwis, on side

Directions:

Place the chicken, broccoli, and beans over the warm rice in small bowl. Top with avocado and hot sauce.

Serve with the kiwis on the side.

NUTRITION (with 2 kiwis, per meal plan): 430 calories, 8 g fat, 1 g sat fat, 58 g carbs, 15 g fiber, 15 g sugar, 37 g protein

EXCHANGES: 2 starches, 4 protein, 1 fruit, 1 vegetable, 1 fat

Chicken Bean Lettuce Wraps (Build Day 14)

4 Bibb or romaine lettuce leaves
1 cup sliced bell peppers
3 ounces grilled chicken breast, sliced
⅓ cup cooked black beans
¼ cup salsa
1 cup raw carrots, on side
½ cup cherry tomatoes, on side
2 tablespoons hummus, on side
1 cup chopped cantaloupe, on side

Directions:

Place two lettuce leaves together on a plate. Top with half the peppers, half the chicken, half the beans, and half the salsa. Repeat with the other two lettuce leaves.

Serve with the carrots, tomatoes, hummus, and cantaloupe on the side.

NUTRITION (with cantaloupe, per meal plan): 420 calories, 8 g fat, 1.5 g sat fat, 59 g carbs, 15 g fiber, 30 g sugar, 38 g protein

EXCHANGES: 1 starch, 4 protein, 1 fruit, 3 vegetables, 1 fat

Chicken Caprese Wrap (Burn Day 11)

2 ounces cooked chicken breast, shredded or chopped
½ cup cherry tomatoes, sliced in half
1 cup chopped romaine lettuce leaves

1 8-inch whole wheat tortilla
1 ounce sliced fresh mozzarella cheese
3 fresh basil leaves, finely chopped
2 teaspoons balsamic vinegar
1 cup grapes, on side

Directions:

Place the chicken, tomatoes, and lettuce on the tortilla. Top with mozzarella, basil, and vinegar. Roll up.

Serve with the grapes on the side.

NUTRITION (with grapes, per the meal plan): 390 calories, 13 g fat, 5 g sat fat, 44 g carbs, 6 g fiber, 19 g sugar, 28 g protein

EXCHANGES: 1½ starches, 2 protein, 1 dairy, 1 fruit, 2 vegetables

Chicken Caesar Wrap (Burn Day 9)

3 ounces cooked chicken breast, shredded or chopped
1 cup chopped romaine lettuce leaves
½ cup cherry tomatoes
1 8-inch whole wheat tortilla
1 tablespoon Parmesan cheese
1 teaspoon olive oil
½ cup raw carrots, on side
1 small orange, on side

Directions:

Place the chicken, romaine, and tomatoes in the tortilla. Top with the Parmesan and oil. Roll up.

Serve with the carrots and orange on the side.

NUTRITION (with carrots and orange, per meal plan): 420 calories, 13 g fat, 3.5 g sat fat, 44 g carbs, 9 g fiber, 15 g sugar, 35 g protein

EXCHANGES: 1½ starches, 3 protein, 1 fruit, 1½ vegetable, 1 fat

Chicken Fajitas (Burn Day 21)

1 teaspoon canola oil
3 ounces chicken breast, raw
¾ cup sliced bell peppers
¾ cup sliced onions
1 8-inch whole wheat tortilla or 2 6-inch corn
    tortillas
¼ cup salsa

Directions:

Heat the oil in a medium skillet over medium-high heat. Add the chicken and sauté for approximately 10 minutes. Add the peppers and onion to the pan (spray with cooking spray, if needed), and sauté for about 10 additional minutes, tossing as needed, until the vegetables are tender and chicken reaches 165 degrees F.

Place the chicken and vegetable mixture onto the tortilla and top with the salsa.

———

NUTRITION: 330 calories, 10 g fat, 2 g sat fat, 38 g carbs, 6 g fiber, 9 g sugar, 26 g protein
EXCHANGES: 1½ starches, 3 protein, 2½ vegetables, 1 fat

Chicken Salad with Quinoa, Cucumber, and Strawberries (Build Day 16)

2 cups spinach leaves
4 ounces cooked chicken breast, shredded or
    chopped
½ cup cooked quinoa
¾ cup sliced cucumbers
¾ cup sliced radishes
½ cup sliced strawberries
1 teaspoon olive oil
2 teaspoons balsamic vinegar

Directions:

Place the spinach in medium bowl. Top with the chicken, quinoa, cucumbers, radishes, and strawberries. Drizzle with the oil and vinegar.

NUTRITION: 410 calories, 12 g fat, 2 g sat fat, 42 g carbs, 8 g fiber, 9 g sugar, 42 g protein
EXCHANGES: 1½ starch, 4 protein, 1 fruit, 2½ vegetables, 1 fat

Chicken "Tacos" (Build Day 20)

The chicken is the taco shell! This is quick, tasty, and full of protein.

1 4-ounce chicken breast, raw
1 tablespoon vegan mayo
¼ avocado, chopped
½ cup bean sprouts
Cayenne pepper, to taste
Greek pepperoncini, to taste

Directions:

Pound the chicken breast thin. Cook over medium heat until done through. Spread the chicken with the vegan mayo. Place all other ingredients on the chicken and fold as a wrap.

———

NUTRITION: 310 calories, 19 g fat, 3 g sat fat, 9 g carbs, 4 g fiber, 3 g sugar, 29 g protein
EXCHANGES: 4 protein, ½ vegetable, 2 fats

Chicken and Vegetable Kabobs with Tzatziki + Rice (Burn Day 17)

3 ounces chopped cooked chicken breast
1 cup bell peppers, chopped in large pieces
½ cup cherry tomatoes
½ cup onions, chopped in large pieces
2 teaspoons canola oil
6 ounces plain fat-free Greek yogurt
2 teaspoons minced garlic
1 tablespoon minced fresh dill
2 teaspoons red wine vinegar
⅓ cup cooked brown rice

Directions:

Preheat the grill to medium-high heat. Alternate placing the chicken, peppers, tomatoes, and onions evenly on two skewers. Brush kabobs with the oil. Grill for approximately 20 minutes, turning occasionally, until chicken reaches 165 degrees F. In a small bowl, mix together the yogurt, garlic, dill, and vinegar to serve as dipping sauce for kabobs.

Serve with the brown rice.

NUTRITION: 450 calories, 13 g fat, 2 g sat fat, 36 g carbs, 5 g fiber, 14 g sugar, 48 g protein
EXCHANGES: 1 starch, 1 dairy, 3 protein, 2 vegetables, 2 fats

Chicken Veggie Pasta (Burn Day 19)

½ cup asparagus, cut into 1-inch pieces
1 teaspoon canola oil
½ cup chopped onion
1 teaspoon minced garlic
½ cup halved cherry tomatoes
3 ounces baked chicken, cut into bite-sized pieces
¾ cup cooked whole wheat fettuccine
1 teaspoon dried oregano
Salt and pepper to taste
1 teaspoon lemon juice
1 teaspoon grated Parmesan cheese

Directions:

Grill or steam the asparagus. Heat the oil in a large pan over medium-high heat. Sauté the onion and garlic for 5–10 minutes or tender. Add the cooked asparagus and raw tomatoes to the pan with the onion and garlic. Cook for approximately 2 minutes or until the tomatoes soften. Add the remaining ingredients and stir until well mixed. Remove from the heat and enjoy.

NUTRITION: 390 calories, 9 g fat, 1.5 g sat fat, 43 g carbs, 9 g fiber, 8 g sugar, 36 g protein
EXCHANGES: 1½ starches, 3 protein, 1½ vegetables, 1 fat

Curried Cauliflower Soup (Cleanse)

This soup serves eight, with approximately 1½ cups of soup per serving. This tastes great with seafood such as grilled shrimp or seared scallops, if you want to add additional protein.

SOUP:

2 heads cauliflower, cored and sliced
6 garlic cloves, sliced
1½ cups chopped white onion (about one large onion)
1½ tablespoons curry powder
1 tablespoon olive oil
½ cup coconut milk
4 cups vegetable stock
Kosher salt, to taste

GARNISH:

1 tablespoon small cauliflower florets
1 teaspoon olive oil
1 teaspoon toasted pine nuts
½ teaspoon chopped parsley
½ teaspoon lemon zest
2 teaspoons golden raisins
Kosher salt, to taste

Directions:

For the Soup:

In a large soup pot, sauté the cauliflower, garlic, onion, and curry powder in the olive oil. Cook on medium heat until the cauliflower starts to become tender. Deglaze the pot with the coconut milk, simmer for about 3 minutes, then add the vegetable stock. Simmer for approximately 30 minutes. Transfer to a blender and blend until smooth, add salt to taste, then pass through a fine-mesh strainer before serving with the garnish.

For the Garnish:

Sauté the cauliflower florets in the olive oil on medium heat until they are evenly golden brown. Turn the heat off, add the pine nuts, parsley, lemon zest, and golden raisins. Season with a pinch of salt, and toss gently.

NUTRITION: 103 calories, 6 g fat, 3.5 g sat fat, 11 g carbs, 4 g fiber, 5 g sugar, 3½ g protein
EXCHANGES: 2 vegetables, 1 fat

Fajita Salad (Build Day 8)

1 teaspoon canola oil
½ cup sliced onion
1 cup sliced bell peppers
2 6-inch corn tortillas, cut into strips
2 cups chopped romaine lettuce leaves
4–5 ounces sliced cooked chicken breast
¼ cup salsa

Directions:

Heat the oil in medium skillet over medium-high heat. Sauté the onions and bell peppers until tender. Preheat the oven to 350 degrees F. Place the tortilla strips on a sheet pan and bake for about 5 minutes or until crisp and slightly golden-brown. Place the romaine in a medium bowl and top with the chicken, sautéed vegetables, and corn tortillas. Stir the salsa into the salad.

NUTRITION: 400 calories, 11 g fat, 2 g sat fat, 37 g carbs, 8 g fiber, 12 g sugar, 40 g protein
EXCHANGES: 1 starch, 4 protein, 3½ vegetables, 1 fat

Greek Chicken and Veggie Pita Pocket (Burn Day 19)

3 ounces chicken breast
Salt and pepper, to taste
2 tablespoons hummus
½ whole wheat pita bread pocket
¼ cup shredded carrots
¼ cup chopped red bell pepper
1 cup sliced cucumbers, on side
2 clementines, on side

Directions:

Preheat the oven to 400 degrees F. Place the chicken on sheet pan and season with salt and pepper to taste. Bake for 20–25 minutes or until the chicken reaches 165 degrees F. Let the chicken sit for 5 minutes, then cut into 1-inch slices. (You can prepare the chicken ahead of time to make this lunch super quick.) Spread the hummus into the pita pocket. Place the chicken, carrots, and bell pepper into pita pocket.

Serve with cucumbers and clementines on the side.

NUTRITION (with cucumbers and clementines, per meal plan): 340 calories, 6 g fat, 2 g sat fat, 49 g carbs, 9 g fiber, 19 g sugar, 28 g protein
EXCHANGES: 1 starch, 3 protein, 1 fruit, 1½ vegetables, 1 fat

Greek Chicken Salad (Build Day 18)

2 cups chopped romaine lettuce leaves
½ cup halved cherry tomatoes
½ cup chopped cucumber
¼ cup crumbled feta cheese
3 ounces baked chicken breast, sliced
1 teaspoon olive oil
1 tablespoon balsamic vinegar
Salt and pepper to taste

Directions:

Top the lettuce with the tomatoes, cucumbers, feta, and chicken. In a small bowl, whisk together the oil, vinegar, and salt and pepper, to taste. Drizzle onto the salad.

NUTRITION: 328 calories, 16 g fat, 7 g sat fat, 12 g carbs, 3 g fiber, 8 g sugar, 34 g protein
EXCHANGES: 3 protein, 1 dairy, 2 vegetables, 1 fat

Jessie's Green Scramble

I make a lot of scrambles, and this is a great one packed with protein! This really gets you fueled up.

2 whole eggs
3 egg whites
1 teaspoon coconut or walnut oil
½ bell pepper, chopped
2 slices cooked turkey (you could use about 1 ounce of cooked chicken if you prefer)
⅓ avocado, sliced
Tomatillo (Mexican green tomato), chopped, to taste
Cayenne pepper, to taste

Beat the whole eggs and egg whites together in a small bowl. Set aside. Heat the oil in a small skillet over medium-high heat. Add the bell pepper, turkey, avocado, and tomatillo and cook until the bell pepper has softened. Add eggs, season with cayenne, and continue to cook on a low heat until the eggs are set the way you like them.

NUTRITION: 392 calories, 23 g fat, 8 g sat fat, 11 g carbs, 6 g fiber, 5 g sugar, 31 g protein
EXCHANGES: 4½ protein, 2 vegetables, 2½ fats

Ham and Veggie Scramble and Toast (Build Day 20)

1 whole egg
2 egg whites
1 cup nonstarchy vegetables (mushrooms, pepper, tomatoes)
1 ounce diced lean ham
2 tablespoons shredded reduced-fat cheddar
1 piece whole wheat toast, on side
1 tablespoon smashed avocado, on side
1 cup chopped honeydew melon, on side

Directions:
Beat the whole egg and egg whites together in small bowl. Set aside. Heat a small skillet over medium-high heat and coat with cooking spray. Sauté the vegetables for about 3–4 minutes or

until crisp-tender. Add the ham and sauté for an additional minute.

Pour in the eggs and cook for approximately 3 minutes or to almost your desired degree of doneness, stirring frequently. Add the cheese and cook for about 30 seconds or until the cheese is melted.

Spread the avocado on the toast, and serve the scramble with the toast and honeydew on the side.

NUTRITION (with toast and melon, per meal plan): 370 calories, 11 g fat, 3.5 g sat fat, 36 g carbs, 6 g fiber, 20 g sugar, 32 g protein
EXCHANGES: 1 starch, 3 protein, ½ dairy, 1 fruit, 1 vegetable, ½ fat

Kale and Chicken Scramble

1 teaspoon coconut or walnut oil
2 slices cooked chicken, chopped
¼ avocado
2 cups raw kale or spinach
2 whole eggs
2 egg whites

Heat the oil in a medium skillet over medium-high heat. Add the chicken, avocado, and kale, and cook until the kale has softened. Scramble the eggs, add them to the pan, and continue to cook on a low heat until set to your liking.

NUTRITION: 410 calories, 23 g fat, 8 g sat fat, 19 g carbs, 6 g fiber, 1 g sugar, 34 g protein
EXCHANGES: 4 protein, 1 vegetable, 2½ fats

Mexican Scramble Soft Tacos (Burn Day 5)

1 teaspoon coconut oil
½ cup chopped red bell pepper
½ cup chopped onion
2 ounces (2–4 slices) chopped turkey (antibiotic-free, nitrate/nitrite-free preferred)
2 tablespoons chopped avocado
1 whole egg

2 egg whites
2 small corn tortillas
Cayenne pepper, to taste
Salt and pepper, to taste

Directions:

Heat the oil in a medium skillet over medium-high heat. Add the bell pepper and onion, and sauté for 4 minutes. Add the turkey and avocado, and sauté for 1 minute. Beat the egg and egg whites together. Mix in the cayenne and salt and pepper to taste. Reduce the heat to medium and add the eggs to the pan. Cook for about 3 minutes, stirring often. Warm corn tortillas for 20 seconds in small skillet or microwave for 10 seconds. Place scramble in tortillas.

NUTRITION: 410 calories, 13 g fat, 6 g sat fat, 43 g carbs, 7 g fiber, 8 g sugar, 30 g protein.
EXCHANGES: 1½ starches, 4 protein, 1 vegetable, 2 fats

Mushroom and Bok Choy Soup (Cleanse)

This soup serves six, with approximately 2 cups of soup per serving. You can substitute other types of mushrooms if you like them, but I encourage you to try these, which have a nice earthy flavor. The soup will taste different if you use other kinds of mushrooms, but you can experiment. If you want additional protein, this soup tastes great with shredded chicken or lentils.

1 red onion, chopped
6 garlic cloves, whole
4 cups cremini mushrooms, stems separated, tops sliced
2 cups shitake mushrooms, stems separated, tops sliced
1 bunch scallions, tops and bulbs separated, finely chopped
1 jalapeño pepper, halved
1 bunch cilantro stems (cut from the bottom of the bunch)
1 tablespoon olive oil

½ cup low-sodium soy sauce
8 cups vegetable stock
4 garlic cloves, minced
8 cups of mushroom-soy broth
2 roasted red peppers, deseeded and julienned into 1-inch pieces
4 cups baby bok choy, thinly sliced, with their tops

Directions:

Brown the onions, whole garlic cloves, cremini mushroom stems, shiitake mushroom stems, scallion bulbs, jalapeño, and cilantro stems in the olive oil over medium-high heat, stirring constantly. Once this mixture is caramelized, add the soy sauce and vegetable stock, and simmer for 30 minutes. Strain the broth and set it aside. Sauté the cremini mushroom tops, shiitake mushroom tops, minced garlic, and scallion tops until the mushrooms become tender (they should not be brown, just soft). Pour in the broth and let it simmer for 20 minutes. Add the roasted peppers and bok choy, cover with a lid, and turn the heat off. Let the soup steep in place with the heat off for about 10 minutes.

NUTRITION: 104 calories, 2.5 g fat, 12½ g carbs, 2½ g fiber, 4½ g sugar, 6 grams protein
EXCHANGES: ½ fat, 3 vegetables, 1 protein

Nut and Berry Cereal Parfait + Hard-Boiled Eggs (Burn Day 21)

You can hard-boil a few eggs in advance to have on hand to add an easy protein boost to your meals when you need them.

1 cup plain fat-free Greek yogurt
½ cup high-fiber cereal, such as shredded wheat
½ cup blueberries
1 tablespoon chopped almonds
Ground cinnamon, to taste
Stevia, to taste (if desired)
1 hard-boiled egg plus hard-boiled egg white, on side

Directions:

Place the yogurt in a small bowl. Top with the cereal, blueberries, almonds, cinnamon, and stevia, if desired.

Serve with the hard-boiled egg and egg white on the side.

NUTRITION (with egg, per meal plan): 370 calories, 10 g fat, 2 g sat fat, 42 g carbs, 6 g fiber, 17 g sugar, 31 g protein
EXCHANGES: 1 starch, 1+ dairy, 1½ protein, ½ fruit, 1 fat

Oatmeal Breakfast Cookies (Burn Day 9)

These can stick to the pan since they don't have butter like regular cookies, so be sure to use a light spray or swipe of oil.

¼ cup + 2 tablespoons uncooked whole rolled oats
½ medium banana, mashed
2 egg whites, lightly beaten
2 teaspoons ground cinnamon
2 tablespoons chopped walnuts

Directions:

Preheat the oven to 375 degrees F. Spray a cookie sheet with cooking spray. Combine all ingredients in a small bowl, and stir until combined. Form the mixture into two small cookies and place on the cookie sheet. Bake for 8–9 minutes or until lightly golden.

NUTRITION: 310 calories, 13 g fat, 1.5 g sat fat, 40 g carbs, 8 g fiber, 8 g sugar, 14 g protein
EXCHANGES: 1½ starches, 2 protein, 1 fruit, 2 fats

Oatmeal Chia Porridge (Burn Day 7)

This is an easy, hearty breakfast, and you do all the work the night before, so it's quick in the morning.

⅓ cup whole rolled oats
1 tablespoon chia seeds
1 cup fat-free or reduced-fat milk
1 scoop whey protein powder
½ cup blueberries
1 teaspoon ground cinnamon

Directions:

Combine the oats, chia seeds, and milk in a small bowl. Cover, and allow to sit in the refrigerator overnight, or at least 8 hours. When ready to eat, stir in the protein powder, and top with the blueberries and cinnamon.

NUTRITION: 410 calories, 9 g fat, 2.5 g sat fat, 52 g carbs, 23 g sugar, 10 g fiber, 32 g protein
EXCHANGES: 1½ starch, 1 dairy, 3 protein, ½ fruit, 1 fat

Peanut Butter/Berry/Egg White Oatmeal (Burn Day 13)

½ cup whole rolled oats
½ cup water
3 egg whites
1 tablespoon natural peanut butter
½ cup blueberries
Ground cinnamon, to taste

Directions:

Mix together the oats, water, and egg whites in small bowl. Cook in a small saucepan on the stove over medium heat for approximately 5 minutes, until the oatmeal reaches your desired consistency. Add more water, if necessary. Alternatively, you can cook this in the microwave on high for 2½–3 minutes (this is one recipe that actually works just fine in the microwave). Mix in the peanut butter, and top with the blueberries and cinnamon.

NUTRITION: 350 calories, 11 g fat, 2 g sat fat, 42 g carbs, 7 g fiber, 10 g sugar, 20 g protein
EXCHANGES: 2 starches, 1½ protein, 1 fruit, 2 fats

Baked Pork Chop with Roasted Sweet Potato and Brussels Sprouts (Burn Day 7)

Everything for this meal can be cooked in one oven, and you've got a great dinner in about 30 minutes.

3 ounces center-cut pork chop, fat trimmed
⅔ sweet potato, chopped
1½ cups Brussels sprouts, halved
1 teaspoon canola oil

Directions:

Preheat the oven to 400 degrees F. Place the pork chop in a pan. Toss the sweet potato pieces and Brussels sprouts in the oil and place on a sheet pan. Place both pans in the oven. Bake for 25–30 minutes, until the pork chop reaches an internal temperature of 145 degrees F and the sweet potato is tender.

NUTRITION: 290 calories, 10 g fat, 2 g sat fat, 27 g carbs, 8 g fiber, 7 g sugar, 21 g protein
EXCHANGES: 1½ starches, 3 protein, 1½ vegetables, 1 fat

Portobello Beef Burger and Zucchini Fries with Marinara Sauce (Build Day 20)

BURGERS:

4 ounces 95% lean ground beef
1 teaspoon garlic powder
Salt and pepper, to taste
2 portobello mushroom caps, gills and stems removed
2 slices avocado
¼ cup arugula
1–2 tomato slices

ZUCCHINI FRIES:

¼ cup panko breadcrumbs
1 teaspoon dried oregano
Salt and pepper, to taste
1 zucchini, cut into approximately 3-inch strips
1 egg white, lightly beaten
⅓ cup marinara sauce (homemade or store-bought)

Directions:

For the Burgers:
Preheat the grill or heat a grill pan over medium-high heat. Mix the beef with the garlic powder and salt and pepper, and form into one patty.

Spray the grill with cooking spray, and grill the mushrooms for about 4 minutes on each side. Keep warm.

Spray the grill with cooking spray again, and grill the ground beef patty for about 3 minutes on each side, or until it reaches the desired degree of doneness.

Place the burger on one of the mushroom caps, top it with the avocado, arugula, tomato, and other mushroom cap.

For the Zucchini Fries:
Preheat the oven to 400 degrees F. Combine the panko, oregano, and salt and pepper in a shallow dish. Dip the zucchini strips into the beaten egg white and lightly dredge each one in the panko mixture. Place on a baking sheet coated with cooking spray.

Bake for 20–25 minutes or until golden brown. Heat the marinara sauce in the microwave or on the stovetop to serve with the zucchini.

NUTRITION: 410 calories, 13 g fat, 3 g sat fat, 42 g carbs, 9 g fiber, 15 g sugar, 36 g protein
EXCHANGES: 1 starch, 4½ protein, 4 vegetables, 1 fat

Power Protein Pancakes
(Build Day 6)

½ cup plain fat-free Greek yogurt
⅓ cup quick-cooking rolled oats
1 whole egg
½ scoop protein powder
2 teaspoons ground cinnamon
½ cup blueberries

Directions:

In a small bowl, stir together all the ingredients except the blueberries until combined.

Heat a medium skillet over medium-high heat. Coat the pan with cooking spray, and pour the batter into the pan to form one large pancake. Cook 3 minutes, flip, and cook an additional 2–3 minutes on the other side. Top with the blueberries and enjoy.

NUTRITION: 350 calories, 8 g fat, 2 g sat fat, 40 g carbs, 8 g fiber, 14 g sugar, 32 g protein
EXCHANGES: 1½ starch, ½ dairy, 2½ protein, ½ fruit

Quinoa Chicken Salad
(Build Day 6)

2 cups chopped romaine lettuce leaves
½ cup cooked quinoa
4 ounces cooked chicken breast, shredded or chopped
½ cup cherry tomatoes
½ cup sliced bell peppers
1 teaspoon olive oil
1 teaspoon balsamic vinegar
1 small peach, on side

Directions:

Place the romaine in medium bowl and top with the quinoa, chicken, tomatoes, and peppers. Drizzle with the oil and vinegar.

Serve with the peach on the side.

NUTRITION (with peach, per meal plan): 410 calories, 11 g fat, 2 sat fat, 36 g carbs, 7 g fiber, 11 g sugar, 42 g protein
EXCHANGES: 1½ starch, 4 protein, 1 fruit, 2 vegetables, 1 fat

Salmon Cakes with Dill Sauce
and Roasted Asparagus
(Build Day 14)

SALMON CAKES:

4 ounces canned or cooked salmon
¼ cup panko breadcrumbs
2 tablespoons diced red bell pepper
1 tablespoon diced celery
2 teaspoons thinly sliced scallion
1 teaspoon lemon juice
½ teaspoon minced garlic
2 tablespoons plain fat-free Greek yogurt
Cayenne pepper, to taste
¼ teaspoon salt and pepper

DILL SAUCE:

½ cup plain fat-free Greek yogurt
1 tablespoon minced fresh dill or
    1½ teaspoons dried dill
1 teaspoon lemon juice

ASPARAGUS:

8–10 stalks asparagus
1 teaspoon canola oil
¼ teaspoon minced garlic
Salt and pepper, to taste

Directions:

For the Salmon Cakes:
Preheat the oven to 425 degrees F. In a medium bowl, flake the salmon to desired size, mix with all other ingredients and stir until combined. Form into two patties and place on a baking sheet coated with cooking spray. Bake for 12–15 minutes.

For the Dill Sauce:
Whisk together the yogurt, dill, and lemon juice.

For the Asparagus:
Place the asparagus on a baking sheet and lightly toss with the oil, garlic, and salt and pepper. Bake at 425 degrees F for about 12–15 minutes or until crisp tender.

NUTRITION: 440 calories, 14 g fat, 2 g sat fat, 31 g carbs, 5 g fiber, 10 g sugar, 47 g protein
EXCHANGES: 1 starch, ½ dairy, 4 protein, 3 vegetables, 1 fat

Salmon, Roasted Beet, and Goat Cheese Salad for Two (Build Day 10)

Serves 2

- 2 small beets (or 1 large beet)
- 2 teaspoons olive oil, divided use
- 1 8-ounce salmon fillet, cut into 2 pieces
- Salt and pepper, to taste
- Juice of ½ lemon
- ½ teaspoon Dijon mustard
- ¼ teaspoon minced garlic
- 4 cups spring mix lettuce
- ½ cup sliced cucumbers
- ½ cup sliced radishes
- 2 tablespoons crumbled goat cheese

Directions:

Clean and slice the beets. Toss with 1 teaspoon of the olive oil and bake for 30–40 minutes at 400 degrees F, flipping once.

Heat a medium sauté pan over medium-high heat and sprinkle the salmon with salt and pepper. Spray the pan with cooking spray and cook the salmon for about 3–4 minutes on each side or until it reaches the desired doneness.

Stir together the lemon juice, mustard, and garlic. Slowly whisk in the remaining 1 teaspoon of olive oil. Add salt and pepper to taste. Set aside.

Toss the the spring mix, cucumbers, radishes, and goat cheese with the dressing. Divide between two plates. Top with the salmon.

Serve with the dressing on the side.

NUTRITION (per serving): 310 calories, 16 g fat, 5 g sat fat, 15 g carbs, 5 g fiber, 7 g sugar, 29 g protein

EXCHANGES (per serving): 4 protein, ½ dairy, 2 vegetables, 1 fat

Salmon Salad Lettuce Wraps (Build Day 16)

- 3 ounces canned salmon
- ¼ cup plain fat-free Greek yogurt
- 2 tablespoons chopped avocado
- ½ cup chopped celery
- 1 teaspoon lemon juice
- Salt and pepper, to taste
- ⅓ cup cooked brown rice
- 4 Bibb lettuce leaves
- 1 cup grapes, on side
- ½ cup baby carrots, on side

Directions:

In a small bowl, mix together the salmon, yogurt, avocado, celery, lemon juice, and salt and pepper.

Spoon the rice evenly into the lettuce leaves, top with the salmon mixture, and enjoy with the grapes and carrots on the side.

NUTRITION (with grapes and carrots, per meal plan): 350 calories, 8 g fat, 1 g sat fat, 43 g carbs, 6 g fiber, 22 g sugar, 30 g protein
EXCHANGES: 1 starch, 3 protein, ⅓ dairy, 1 fruit, 1½ vegetables, 1 fat

Shrimp Sautéed with Broccoli and Rice (Burn Day 11)

- 1½ cups broccoli florets
- 1 teaspoon canola oil
- 3–5 ounces medium shrimp, peeled and deveined
- 2 tablespoons Parmesan cheese
- ½ cup cooked brown rice

Directions:

Steam the broccoli florets for 5–6 minutes, or until crisp-tender. Set aside.

Heat the oil in a medium skillet over medium-high heat. Add the shrimp and broccoli and sauté for about 3–5 minutes, or until the shrimp are thoroughly cooked. Sprinkle with the Parmesan.

Serve with the rice.

NUTRITION: 300 calories, 10 g fat, 2.5 g sat fat, 29 g carbs, 5 g fiber, 0 g sugar, 25 g protein
EXCHANGES: 1½ starches, 4 protein, ½ dairy, 1½ vegetables, 1 fat

Shrimp Stir-Fry (Burn Day 5)

1 tablespoon water
1 tablespoon low-sodium soy sauce
¼ teaspoon garlic powder
¼ teaspoon ground ginger
1 teaspoon cornstarch
2 teaspoons canola oil
2 cups raw nonstarchy vegetables of your choice (broccoli, mushrooms, bell peppers, onions)
3 ounces medium shrimp, peeled and deveined
1 cup cooked soba noodles

Directions:

In a small bowl, mix the soy sauce, water, garlic powder, ginger, and cornstarch together.

Heat the oil in a large skillet over medium-high heat. Add the vegetables and sauté for about 8–10 minutes, or until crisp-tender.

Add the shrimp to the pan and continue sautéing for 3–4 minutes or until the shrimp are cooked thoroughly.

Mix the noodles with the soy sauce mixture, add to the pan, and stir over the heat for 1–2 minutes.

NUTRITION: 340 calories, 11 g fat, 2 g sat fat, 43 g carbs, 4 g fiber, 5 g sugar, 22 g protein
EXCHANGES: 2 starches, 3 protein, 2 vegetables, 2 fats

SMOOTHIES

You can use whatever type of protein powder you prefer in any of the smoothies. I recommend whey-, pea-, or hemp-based powders as a first choice.

Green Tea Smoothie (for Cleanse Days)

1 cup brewed green tea, cooled
1 scoop protein powder
½ medium banana
1 tablespoon lemon juice
1 tablespoon ground flaxseed
1 cup spinach

Directions:

Blend all ingredients with ice to taste.

NUTRITION: 200 calories, 4 g fat, 1 g sat fat, 20 g carbs, 4 g fiber, 9 g sugar, 24 g protein
EXCHANGES: 3 protein, 1 fruit, ½ vegetable, 1 fat

Upgraded Green Tea Smoothie (for Burn/Build Days)

1 cup brewed green tea, cooled
1 scoop protein powder
1 medium banana
1 tablespoon lemon juice
2 tablespoons ground flaxseed
1 cup spinach

Directions:

Blend all ingredients with ice to taste.

NUTRITION: 290 calories, 7 g fat, 1 g sat fat, 36 g carbs, 8 g fiber, 16 g sugar, 26 g protein
EXCHANGES: 3 protein, 2 fruits, ½ vegetable, 2 fats

Chocolate-Covered Strawberry Smoothie (for Cleanse Days)

1 cup plain unsweetened almond milk
1 scoop protein powder
2 tablespoons unsweetened cocoa powder
1 cup sliced strawberries

Directions:
Blend all ingredients with ice to taste.

NUTRITION: 214 calories, 5 g fat, 1 g sat fat, 25 g carbs, 9 g fiber, 10 g sugar, 21 g protein
EXCHANGES: 3 protein, 1 fruit, 1 fat

Upgraded Chocolate-Covered Strawberry Smoothie (for Burn/Build Days)

1 cup plain unsweetened almond milk
1 scoop protein powder
2 tablespoons unsweetened cocoa powder
2 cups sliced strawberries
1 tablespoon chia seeds
1 tablespoon dark chocolate chips
   (>70% cocoa)

Directions:
Blend all ingredients with ice to taste.

NUTRITION: 370 calories, 14 g fat, 4 g sat fat, 45 g carbs, 15 g fiber, 25 g sugar, 25 g protein
EXCHANGES: 3 protein, 2 fruits, 2 fats

Java Mocha Smoothie (for Cleanse Days)

1 cup brewed coffee, cooled
¾ cup plain fat-free Greek yogurt
½ medium banana
1 tablespoon unsweetened cocoa powder
1 tablespoon ground flaxseed

Directions:
Blend all ingredients with ice to taste.

NUTRITION: 192 calories, 4 g fat, .5 g sat fat, 25 g carbs, 6 g fiber, 13 g sugar, 21 g protein
EXCHANGES: 1 dairy, ½ fruit, 1 fat

Upgraded Java Mocha Smoothie (for Burn/Build Days)

1 cup brewed coffee, cooled
1 cup plain fat-free Greek yogurt
1 tablespoon unsweetened cocoa powder
2 tablespoons ground flaxseed
1 medium banana

Directions:
Blend all ingredients with ice to taste. If you peel and chop the banana and freeze it beforehand, you may not want ice at all.

NUTRITION: 310 calories, 6 g fat, .5 g sat fat, 44 g carbs, 9 g fiber, 24 g sugar, 26 g protein
EXCHANGES: 1+ dairy, 2 fruits, 2 fats

Tropical Kale Smoothie (for Cleanse Days)

¾ cup plain fat-free Greek yogurt
½ cup water
½ cup chopped pineapple
1 tablespoon ground flaxseed
1 cup chopped kale

Directions:
Blend all ingredients with ice to taste.

NUTRITION: 200 calories, 3 g fat, 0 g sat fat, 27 g carbs, 4 g fiber, 15 g sugar, 22 g protein
EXCHANGES: 1 dairy, 1 fruit, ½ vegetable, 1 fat

Upgraded Tropical Kale Smoothie (for Burn/Build Days)

1 cup plain fat-free Greek yogurt
½ cup water
1 cup chopped pineapple
1 tablespoon ground flaxseed
1½ cups chopped kale

Directions:

Blend all ingredients with ice to taste.

NUTRITION: 290 calories, 4 g fat, 0 g sat fat, 43 g carbs, 6 g fiber, 24 g sugar, 27 g protein
EXCHANGES: 1+ dairy, 2 fruits, 1 ½ vegetables, 1 fat

Cherry Almond Smoothie (for Cleanse Days)

1 cup plain unsweetened almond milk
¾ cup frozen cherries
1 scoop protein powder
1 cup spinach (optional)

Directions:

Blend all ingredients with ice to taste.

NUTRITION: 220 calories, 4.5 g fat, 1 g sat fat, 23 g carbs, 4 g fiber, 14 g sugar, 24 g protein
EXCHANGES: 3 protein, 1 fruit, ½ vegetable, 1 fat

Upgraded Cherry Almond Smoothie (for Burn/Build Days)

1 cup plain unsweetened almond milk
1½ cups frozen cherries
1 scoop protein powder
1½ cups spinach (optional)
1 tablespoon ground flaxseed

Directions:

Blend all ingredients with ice to taste.

NUTRITION: 330 calories, 7 g fat, 1 g sat fat, 44 g carbs, 9 g fiber, 28 g sugar, 26 g protein
EXCHANGES: 3 protein, 2 fruits, 1 vegetable, 2 fats

Blueberry Pear Smoothie

1 cup fat-free unsweetened kefir
⅓ cup blueberries
⅓ cup chopped pear
1 tablespoon chia seeds
1 cup arugula (optional)

Directions:

Blend all ingredients with ice to taste.

NUTRITION: 211 calories, 3 g fat, 1 g sat fat, 32 g carbs, 8 g fiber, 22 g sugar, 15 g protein
EXCHANGES: 1 dairy, 1 protein, 1 fruit, ½ vegetable, 1 fat

Upgraded Blueberry Pear Smoothie

1 cup fat-free unsweetened kefir
½ cup blueberries
⅔ cup chopped pear
1 tablespoon chia seeds
1½ cups arugula (optional)
½ scoop protein powder

Directions:

Blend all ingredients with ice to taste.

NUTRITION: 320 calories, 4.5 g fat, 1 g sat fat, 46 g carbs, 11 g fiber, 28 g sugar, 28 g protein
EXCHANGES: 1 dairy, 1½ protein, 2 fruits, 1 vegetable, 1 fat

Pumpkin Smoothie

1 cup canned pumpkin (no sugar added)
6 ounces plain fat-free yogurt
1 scoop protein powder
½ cup water
1 tablespoon chopped walnuts
½ teaspoon ground cinnamon
¼ teaspoon ground nutmeg
¼ teaspoon ground cloves
1 stevia packet, if desired

Directions:

Combine all ingredients in a blender and blend until smooth. If you like a thicker consistency, blend with ice to taste.

NUTRITION: 340 calories, 6 g fat, 2 g sat fat, 40 g carbs, 8 g fiber, 22 g sugar, 36 g protein
EXCHANGES: 1 dairy, 3 protein, 1 fruit, 1 fat

Sweet and Spicy Chicken Breast with Mashed Sweet Potatoes and Broccoli (Burn Day 9)

CHICKEN:

1 3-ounce chicken breast
¼ teaspoon dried oregano
¼ teaspoon garlic powder
Dash cayenne pepper (optional)
⅛ teaspoon ground cumin
1 tablespoon honey
½ teaspoon apple cider vinegar

MASHED SWEET POTATOES:

½ small sweet potato, chopped
3 tablespoons plain fat-free Greek yogurt
1 teaspoon garlic powder
Salt and pepper, to taste

BROCCOLI:

1½ cups chopped broccoli
1 teaspoon olive oil
½ teaspoon crushed red pepper
Salt and pepper, to taste

Directions:

For the Chicken:
Preheat the oven to 400 degrees F. Sprinkle the chicken breast with the oregano, garlic, cayenne, and cumin and place on a baking sheet coated with cooking spray. Bake for about 20 minutes, or until the chicken reaches an internal temperature of 165 degrees F. Remove the chicken from the oven.

Mix the honey and vinegar together. Brush or spoon about half the honey mixture on one side of the chicken breast. Return the chicken to the oven and bake for 2 more minutes. Flip the chicken over, put the remaining honey mixture on the chicken, and bake for 2 more minutes.

For the Sweet Potato:
Boil the sweet potato until tender and drain. Place the potato and the remaining ingredients in medium bowl. Blend with a hand mixer or masher until combined to desired consistency.

For the Broccoli:
Toss the broccoli with the oil, crushed red pepper, and salt and pepper. Place on a baking sheet and bake at 400 degrees F for about 10–15 minutes.

NUTRITION: 350 calories, 8 g fat, 1.5 g sat fat, 46 g carbs, 7 g fiber, 23 g sugar, 27 g protein
EXCHANGES: 1½ starch, 3 protein, 1½ vegetables, 1 fat

Tomato-Cucumber Gazpacho (Cleanse)

This refreshing cold soup serves six, with approximately 2 cups per serving. It pairs well with seafood, such as grilled shrimp, scallops, salmon, or even oysters.

- 2 16-ounce cans of San Marzano plum tomatoes in juice, drained (reserve the juice) and diced
- 1½ cucumbers, peeled and cut into small dice
- ¼ red onion, cut into small dice (about ½ cup)
- 1 bunch scallions, tops only, finely chopped
- 1½ tablespoons cilantro, finely chopped
- ¼ cup rice wine vinegar
- 1 tablespoon hot sauce
- Juice of 1 lemon, divided use
- 1 tablespoon kosher salt
- 1 avocado, ripe but firm, cut into small dice
- 1 cup watercress

Directions:

Lightly squeeze the tomatoes to get rid of excess juice, being careful not to damage the tomatoes. Combine the tomatoes, cucumbers, onions, scallions, cilantro, vinegar, hot sauce, all but ½ teaspoon of the lemon juice (reserve the ½ teaspoon for serving), and salt in a large mixing bowl. Add the avocado and mix gently so as to not damage the avocado. Taste, and adjust seasoning if necessary. Use some of the reserved juice from the tomatoes as needed to get the texture you like for this soup. Let the gazpacho marinate overnight for best results. Before serving, toss the watercress with the reserved ½ teaspoon of the lemon juice in a small bowl, and use this to garnish the gazpacho.

NUTRITION: 92 calories, 4 g fat, 12 g carbs, 5 g fiber, 7 g sugar, 3 g protein
EXCHANGES: 1 fat, 2 vegetables

Tortilla Pizza with Green Salad (Burn Day 17)

PIZZA:

- 1 8-inch whole wheat tortilla
- ¼ cup tomato sauce (homemade or from a jar)
- 1 teaspoon dried basil
- ¼ cup shredded reduced-fat mozzarella cheese
- 2 tablespoons chopped deli ham
- ½ cup sliced nonstarchy vegetables (mushrooms, bell pepper, broccoli)

SALAD:

- 2 cups romaine or other lettuce
- ½ cup nonstarchy vegetables
- 1 teaspoon olive oil
- 2 teaspoons balsamic vinegar

Directions:

Preheat the oven to 350 degrees F. Top the tortilla with the tomato sauce, basil, cheese, ham, and vegetables. Bake for 10–12 minutes, until the cheese is bubbling. Meanwhile, toss the lettuce, vegetables, olive oil, and vinegar together to make the salad.

NUTRITION (with salad, per meal plan): 358 calories, 16 g fat, 5 g sat fat, 39 g carbs, 9 g fiber, 8 g sugar, 20 g protein
EXCHANGES: 1½ starches, 2 protein, 1 dairy, 3 vegetables, 1 fat

Tuna Spinach Salad (Build Day 8)

- 2 cups spinach leaves
- ½ cup cherry tomatoes
- 4 ounces canned tuna, drained
- ⅓ cup cooked kidney beans
- 1 teaspoon olive oil
- 2 teaspoons balsamic vinegar
- 1 small pear, on side

Directions:

Place the spinach leaves in a medium bowl, and top with the tomatoes, tuna, and beans. Drizzle the oil and vinegar over the salad.

Serve with the pear on the side.

NUTRITION (with 1 small pear, per meal plan): 390 calories, 9 g fat, 1 g sat fat, 46 g carbs, 12 g fiber, 18 g sugar, 34 g protein
EXCHANGES: 1 starch, 4 protein, 1 fruit, 1½ vegetables, 1 fat

Turkey Burger and Green Salad (Burn Day 21)

BURGER:

3 ounces extra lean ground turkey, formed into a burger patty
1 2-ounce whole wheat bun
2 slices avocado

SALAD:

2 cups greens (such as spinach, romaine, lettuce of your choice)
½ cup cherry tomatoes
½ cup chopped cucumbers
1 teaspoon olive oil
2 teaspoons balsamic vinegar

FRUIT:

2 kiwis, on side

Directions:

Heat a skillet or grill pan over medium-high heat. Coat the pan with cooking spray, and cook the turkey burger 3–4 minutes per side or until the internal temperature reaches 165 degrees F. Place the burger on the bun, and top with the avocado.

Place the greens in a medium bowl, and top with the tomatoes and cucumbers. Drizzle with the oil and vinegar.

Serve with the kiwis on the side.

NUTRITION (with 2 kiwis, per meal plan): 460 calories, 14 g fat, 2 g sat fat, 61 g carbs, 13 g fiber, 23 g sugar, 30 g protein
EXCHANGES: 2 starches, 3 protein, 1 fruit, 2 vegetables, 2 fats

Turkey Meatballs and Marinara with Zucchini Noodles (Build Day 12)

TURKEY MEATBALLS:

4 ounces ground turkey breast
¼ teaspoon dried oregano
½ teaspoon minced garlic
Salt and pepper, to taste
¼ cup panko breadcrumbs

MARINARA:

1 teaspoon canola oil
¼ cup chopped onion
¼ teaspoon minced garlic
1 cup canned crushed tomatoes
Salt and pepper, to taste

ZUCCHINI NOODLES:

2 zucchini
¼ teaspoon minced garlic

Directions:

For the Meatballs and Marinara:

Combine all meatball ingredients in a medium bowl, and stir until well combined. Form into 2–3 meatballs and place in the refrigerator until ready to cook.

In a small saucepan, heat the oil over medium-high heat. Sauté the onion and garlic for 5–7 minutes or until tender. Add the crushed tomatoes, and salt and pepper and reduce the heat to medium.

Place the meatballs into the sauce, cover, and simmer for about 20 minutes or until the meatballs reach 165 degrees F.

For the Zucchini Noodles:

Using a vegetable peeler, peel the zucchini into long strips.

Heat a small skillet over medium-high heat and coat it with cooking spray. Add the zucchini and sauté for about 4–6 minutes or until tender. Stir in the garlic and cook for an additional 30 seconds. Place the meatballs and marinara over the zucchini noodles and enjoy.

NUTRITION: 355 calories, 6 g fat, 1 g sat fat, 40 g carbs, 9 g fiber, 16 g sugar, 36 g protein

EXCHANGES: 1 starch, 4 protein, 4 vegetables, 1 fat

Turkey Mushroom Scramble

1 whole egg
2 egg whites
Salt and pepper, to taste
1 teaspoon coconut oil
1 cup chopped mushrooms of your choice
2 ounces (2–4 slices) turkey, chopped
1 cup spinach leaves
½ English muffin, toasted, on side
1 teaspoon butter (optional), on side

Directions:

Beat the eggs and egg whites together and season with salt and pepper to taste.

Heat the oil in a medium skillet over medium-high heat. Add the mushrooms and turkey and sauté for about 4 minutes. Add the spinach and sauté for about 1 minute, or until it has wilted.

Reduce the heat to medium. Add the eggs to pan and cook for about 3 minutes, stirring often, until you reach desired degree of doneness.

Serve with the toasted English muffin half and butter, if desired.

NUTRITION: 330 calories, 14 g fat, 8 g sat fat, 19 g carbs, 2 g fiber, 2 g sugar, 35 g protein

EXCHANGES: 4 protein, 1½ vegetables, 2 fat, 1 starch

Turkey Taco Wraps and Salad (Build Day 6)

TACOS:

4 ounces ground turkey breast
¼ cup finely chopped red bell pepper
¼ cup finely chopped onion
½ teaspoon minced garlic
Dash cayenne pepper
¼ teaspoon salt and pepper
⅓ cup tomato sauce
3 tablespoons water
4 Bibb or romaine lettuce leaves
2 slices avocado
¼ cup plain fat-free Greek yogurt

SALAD:

2 cups spring mix or other greens of your choice
¼ cup cherry tomatoes
¼ cup chopped red bell pepper
1 teaspoon olive oil
1 tablespoon balsamic vinegar
¼ teaspoon minced garlic
Dash cayenne pepper
Salt and pepper, to taste

Directions:

For the Tacos:

Heat a medium skillet over medium-high heat. Coat the pan with cooking spray and add the turkey, peppers, onion, and garlic. Cook until turkey thoroughly cooked (165 degrees F) and the vegetables are tender.

Mix the cayenne, salt and pepper, tomato sauce, and water together. Add to the skillet and simmer for about 15 minutes or until the sauce is reduced. Place the turkey mixture onto the lettuce and top with the avocado and Greek yogurt.

For the Salad:

Place the spring mix, tomatoes, and bell pepper into small bowl. Whisk together the oil, vinegar, garlic, cayenne, and salt and pepper, and mix into the salad.

NUTRITION: 360 calories, 11 g fat, 1 g sat fat, 32 g carbs, 10 g fiber, 15 g sugar, 40 g protein
EXCHANGES: 4 protein, 4 vegetables, 2 fats

Turkey Wrap with Veggies (Burn Day 13)

¼ cup plain fat-free Greek yogurt
1 tablespoon minced fresh dill
Salt and pepper, to taste
2 ounces cooked turkey
1 ounce reduced-fat Swiss cheese
1 cup spring mix
3 slices tomato
1 tablespoon mustard
1 8-inch whole wheat tortilla
1 small apple, on side
1 cup sliced bell peppers, on side
1 cup sliced cucumbers, on side

Directions:

Mix together the yogurt and dill with salt and pepper to taste. Set aside.

Place the turkey, cheese, spring mix, tomato, and mustard on the tortilla. Roll up.

Serve the wrap with an apple and vegetables with yogurt dip on the side.

NUTRITION (with apple per meal plan): 420 calories, 6 g fat, 1 g sat fat, 58 g carbs, 10 g fiber, 20 g sugar, 27 g protein
EXCHANGES: 1½ starches, 1+ dairy, 2 protein, 1 fruit, 3 vegetables

Crisp Crunchy Vegetable Medley

Give this a try—it's a very satisfying snack! If you haven't tried Himalayan salt yet, please do!

½ cucumber, sliced
¼ onion, sliced
¼ red pepper, sliced
2 radishes, sliced
4 tablespoons apple cider vinegar
Juice of 1 lemon
Himalayan salt, to taste

Directions:

Slice the vegetables into similarly sized pieces. Toss them with the vinegar and lemon juice in a small bowl. Sprinkle with salt to taste.

NUTRITION: 55 calories, 0 g fat, 12 g carbs, 2 g fiber, 7 g sugar, 1 g protein
EXCHANGES: 2 vegetables

Vegetable Broth

You can use this as a base for the other soups or to have on hand for use as a calorie-free snack.

1 gallon (16 cups) tap water
1 large onion, chopped
4 cups celery, chopped
6 garlic cloves, peeled and halved
6 sprigs thyme
1 bunch parsley stems
2 bay leaves
1 teaspoon kosher salt
1 teaspoon black peppercorns

Directions:

Add all ingredients to a large stockpot, and simmer for 1 hour. Strain through a fine-mesh strainer.

Exchanges: You can use the vegetable broth as a "free" food on The Program.

White Bean and Tuscan Kale Soup (Cleanse)

This soup serves eight, with approximately 1½ cups per serving. The soup goes great with diced or shredded chicken as a protein option.

3 cups uncooked white beans
½ yellow onion, chopped into small dice
3 garlic cloves, minced
5 carrots, peeled and diced
1 teaspoon fresh thyme, chopped
1 tablespoon flat leaf parsley, chopped
½ teaspoon fresh rosemary, chopped
1 tablespoon olive oil
½ gallon vegetable broth (see page 212)
1 bay leaf
1 tablespoon kosher salt
3 cups julienned Tuscan kale
½ tablespoon Arugula Pesto Garnish (per portion; see below)

Directions:

Cook the beans in water to cover for approximately 1 hour, or until al dente. Drain them and set aside. In a large soup pot, sauté the onions, garlic, carrots, thyme, parsley, and rosemary in the olive oil. Add the vegetable broth, bay leaf, and salt. Simmer until the carrots become tender. Turn off the heat, and remove the bay leaf. Stir the kale into the hot soup until it becomes blanched and bright green. Add a spoonful of Arugula Pesto as garnish.

NUTRITION: 160 calories, 2 g fat, 28 g carbs, 7 g fiber, 6 g sugar, 8 g protein
EXCHANGES: 1 starch, 1 protein, 2+ vegetables, ½ fat

Arugula Pesto Garnish

Serving size: 1 teaspoon
6 ounces wild arugula
1½ teaspoons toasted pine nuts
1 garlic clove
Juice of ½ lemon
½ teaspoon kosher salt
3 tablespoons olive oil

Directions:

Place all ingredients except the olive oil in a food processor or blender. Blend until mixed, then slowly add the oil until the mixture is thick and emulsified.

NUTRITION: 25 calories, 2½ g fat
EXCHANGES: ½ fat

Build Day Snacks (100–200 calories)

Low-fat string cheese + 100-calorie pack of almonds (180 calories, 12 g protein)

½ cup low-fat cottage cheese + ½ cup raw cherry tomatoes (125 calories, 12 g protein)

½ cup steamed edamame (100 calories, 8 g protein)

2 ounces lean jerky (turkey/bison) (160 calories, 24 g protein)

2 hard-boiled eggs (140 calories, 12 g protein)

2 slices deli meat + 1 slice low-fat cheese roll-up (200 calories, 16 g protein)

6 ounces plain or vanilla fat-free Greek yogurt with 1 tablespoon sunflower seeds (140 calories, 19 g protein)

Mini smoothie: 1 scoop vanilla protein powder + ½ cup frozen berries + 8 ounces water (140 calories, 20 g protein)

Burn Day Snacks (100–200 calories)

Celery sticks + 1 tablespoon natural peanut butter (110 calories, 4 g protein)

¼ cup hummus + 1 cup raw vegetables (160 calories, 7 g protein)

1 cup grapes + 1 ounce low-fat string cheese (130 calories, 9 g protein)

1 small banana + 1 tablespoon natural peanut butter (180 calories, 4 g protein)

Small apple + 1 tablespoon almond butter (160 calories, 5 g protein)

Small pear + 1 ounce low-fat string cheese (160 calories, 9 g protein)

2 small kiwis + 7 walnut halves (180 calories, 4 g protein)

1 small orange + 1 hard-boiled egg (130 calories, 6 g protein)

½ mango + 100-calorie pack of almonds (150 calories, 4 g protein)

6 ounces plain or vanilla fat-free Greek yogurt with ½ cup berries (130 calories, 17 g protein)

Jessie's Favorite Flavor Enhancers

Use these if you're looking to add flavor with very few calories—they can really make a difference and if it helps you increase your fruit and vegetable intake, it's all good!

Apple cider vinegar with the mother
Cayenne pepper
Cinnamon
Turmeric
Fresh lemon juice

Food Exchange Options

I hope that you'll try new foods while you're on The Program, but I have provided food category exchanges in the meal plans so that you can adjust the menus to your taste (or for other people you cook for) and still stick to the ratios for each meal or day. Use the categories below to swap out foods as needed. This list is adapted from the American Dietetic Association Food Exchange Lists, which are available online. The American Diabetes Association also provides a comprehensive list of exchanges you can consult. Note: A "+" sign after an exchange number = slightly more than the allotted number. In some cases smaller quantities of ingredients have not been included in exchanges.

Protein

Very lean protein choices have 35 calories and 1 gram of fat per serving. One serving equals:

- 1 ounce turkey breast or chicken breast, skin removed
- 1 ounce fish fillet (flounder, sole, scrod, cod, etc.)
- 1 ounce canned tuna in water
- 1 ounce shellfish (clams, lobster, scallop, shrimp)
- ¾ cup cottage cheese, nonfat or low-fat (3 proteins)
- ¾ cup plain, nonfat Greek yogurt (3 proteins)
- 2 egg whites
- ¼ cup egg substitute
- 1 ounce fat-free cheese
- ½ cup beans, cooked (black beans, kidney, chickpeas, or lentils; these count as both 1 starch/bread and 1 very lean protein)

Lean protein choices have 55 calories and 2–3 grams of fat per serving. One serving equals:

- 1 ounce chicken (dark meat, skin removed)
- 1 ounce turkey (dark meat, skin removed)
- 1 ounce salmon, swordfish, herring
- 1 ounce lean beef (flank steak, London broil, tenderloin, roast beef)*
- 1 ounce veal, roast or lean chop*
- 1 ounce lamb, roast or lean chop*

1 ounce pork, tenderloin or fresh ham*
1 ounce low-fat cheese (with 3 g or
      less of fat per ounce)
¼ cup 4.5% cottage cheese
2 tablespoons grated Parmesan cheese

* Limit these choices to no more than once or twice a week. Also, when I buy meat, I try to buy organic and nitrate-free when possible.

Medium-fat proteins have 75 calories and 5 grams of fat per serving. One serving equals:

1 ounce beef (any prime cut), corned
      beef, ground beef**
1 ounce pork chop**
1 whole egg (medium)
1 ounce mozzarella cheese
¼ cup ricotta cheese
4 ounces tofu

** Choose these very infrequently

Dairy

Fat-Free and Very Low-Fat Milk contain 90 calories per serving. One serving equals:

1 cup milk, fat-free or 1% fat
¾ cup yogurt, plain nonfat or low-fat
¾ cup plain, nonfat Greek yogurt*
¾ cup kefir
1 ounce cheese
½ cup cottage cheese

Note that the composition of alternative milks made from soy, almond, rice, and so on varies greatly, so if you like these, make sure the protein, carbohydrate, and calcium content are meeting your needs.

* Note that cheese, cottage cheese, and Greek yogurt are considered either protein or dairy. In all of the recipes above they are counted as dairy to keep things simple.

Fruits And Vegetables

Fruits contain 15 grams of carbohydrate and 60 calories. One serving equals:

1 small apple, banana, orange, or
      nectarine
1 medium peach
½ medium banana
1 kiwi
½ grapefruit
¾ cup cherries (fresh or frozen)
½ mango
1 cup strawberries, raspberries, or
      blueberries
1 cup melon cubes
⅛ honeydew melon
4 ounces unsweetened juice*
¼ cup dried fruit*

* I don't recommend too much dried fruit or juice because it's too high in sugar—fresh, whole fruit is always your BEST option.

Vegetables contain 25 calories and 5 grams of carbohydrate. One serving equals:

1 cup cooked or raw vegetables
2 cups raw leafy salad greens
½ cup vegetable juice

If you are hungry while following the meal plans on The Program, eat additional fresh or steamed vegetables! Great nonstarchy vegetable choices include:

Artichokes
Asparagus
Bamboo shoots
Beans (green, wax, Italian)
Bean sprouts
Beets
Bell peppers
Bok choy
Broccoli
Brussels sprouts
Cabbage (all types)
Carrots
Cauliflower
Celery
Coleslaw, no dressing
Cucumber
Eggplant
Endive
Escarole
Greens (collard, kale, mustard, turnip)
Hearts of palm

Jicama
Kohlrabi
Leeks
Lettuce (arugula, radicchio, romaine, Bibb, chicory, endive, watercress)
Mixed vegetables (without corn or peas)
Mung bean sprouts
Mushrooms
Okra
Onions
Salsa (¼ cup)
Sauerkraut
Spinach
Summer Squash
Swiss Chard
Tomatoes
Turnips
Zucchini

Carbohydrates

Starches/carbohydrates contain 15 grams of carbohydrate and 80 calories per serving. One serving equals:

1 slice bread (white, pumpernickel, whole wheat, rye)
¼ bagel (varies by size; one serving is 1 ounce)
½ English muffin
½ hamburger bun
¾ cup dry cereal
¼ cup dry oats (or ½ cup cooked oats)
⅓ cup rice, brown or white, cooked

⅓ cup barley, quinoa, or couscous,
   cooked
⅓ cup dried beans, peas, or lentils,
   cooked
½ cup pasta, cooked
½ cup bulgur wheat, cooked
½ cup corn
½ cup sweet potato
½ cup green peas
3 cups popcorn, hot air popped or
   microwave

Fats

Fats contain 45–50 calories and 5 grams
of fat per serving. One serving equals:

1 teaspoon oil (coconut, walnut,
   vegetable, corn, canola, olive, etc.)

1 teaspoon butter
1 tablespoon seeds (flaxseed,
   pumpkin, sunflower, sesame, chia)
1½ teaspoons nut butter (almond,
   cashew, peanut; choose trans fat–
   free butters)
1 teaspoon mayonnaise (vegan is
   worth trying)
1 tablespoon most salad dressings
⅕ avocado (about 1 ounce) or
   2 tablespoons mashed avocado
8 large black olives
1 slice nitrate-free bacon
2 tablespoons shredded coconut
2 tablespoons hummus

Acknowledgments

Thank you to my mother, Terri, for teaching me what love and compassion are and to my father, Mike, one of the hardest working men I know, who still finds time to chase his dreams. Thank you to my son, Rowan: I had forgotten how important it is to appreciate every minute until you came into my life. I am continually inspired by the experiences and courage of the amazing people I have trained and grateful for everything they teach me, especially about how important it is to listen and to believe in yourself. A special thanks to Stacy Creamer at Hachette Books, for believing in me and what I do; to Melissa Moore, one rad writer; and to Dr. Melina Jampolis, Ashley Marriott, and my team Jill Tipping, Ryan Haden, Scott Howard, and Richard Abate for their help with The Program.

Index